Marcel Paraschivescu
Marcel Theodor Paraschivescu

AF155870

Undemonstrative Outputs of Sheep Breeding Disclosed by Biotechnologies

LAP LAMBERT Academic Publishing

Publisher:
LAP LAMBERT Academic Publishing
is a trademark of
Dodo Books Indian Ocean Ltd. and OmniScriptum S.R.L publishing group

120 High Road, East Finchley, London, N2 9ED, United Kingdom
Str. Armeneasca 28/1, office 1, Chisinau MD-2012, Republic of Moldova, Europe
Managing Directors: Ieva Konstantinova, Victoria Ursu
info@omniscriptum.com

Printed at: see last page
ISBN: 978-3-659-56552-6

Marcel Paraschivescu
Marcel Theodor Paraschivescu

Undemonstrative Outputs of Sheep Breeding Disclosed by Biotechnologies

TABLE OF CONTENTS

FOREWORD 3

INTRODUCTION 5

Chapter 1
THE GENETIC SPECIES OF SHEEP AND ITS BIODIVERSITY .. 7

Biological diversity concept 7

Biodiversity in sheep 9

Identity in biological diversity of sheep 14

Chapter 2
PARTICULARITIES OF REPRODUCTION IN SHEEP 18

Reproduction seasonality 18

Lambing interval and the fertility in sheep 22

Reproduction Systems 24

Chapter 3
BIOTECHNOLOGICAL PROCEDURES IN SHEEP REPRODUCTION 27

Reproduction biotechnologies concerning the male side 27

Biotechnologies concerning the female side 29

Additional means to help estrous synchronization in ewes 42

Estrous synchronization outside of the mating season 46

In vitro fertilization (IVF) and advanced genomic biotechnologies 49

Chapter 4
DISCLOSING OUTPUTS OF SHEEP BREEDING BY BIOTECHNOLOGIES 52

Concept 52

Getting genetic progress of breeding stock 55

Increasing the commercial value of farm outputs 56

Ex situ biodiversity preservation 60

Chapter 5
VIRTUES AND SERVITUDES OF BREEDING BIOTECHNOLOGY IN SHEEP (Instead of conclusions) 64

Future of biotechnologies in sheep breeding 64

Future of biodiversity in sheep farming 69

BIBLIOGRAPHY 71

FOREWORD

This book is due to the project number POSDRU/89/1.5/S/ 63258 "Postdoctoral school for farm animal biodiversity and food biotechnology based on the eco-economy and the bio-economy required by eco sanogenesis", co-financed from the European Social Fund through Sectorial Operational Programmed Human Resources Development 2007-2013, where I have been one of the students and had to prepare the postdoctoral thesis "MOET Virtues and Servitudes in Farm Animal Species Related to Their Biodiversity" as theoretical extension of my PhD thesis "Project study to foundation of an open MOET farm in dairy cattle".[1] But the merit of publishing this book belongs to LAP LAMBERT Academic Publishing, a trademark of *Omni Scriptum* GmbH & Co. KG and to its Iuliana Oaserele Acquisition Editor. They have selected the title from a report concerning results of the above mentioned project and made the offer to finance and publish it.

As I have mentioned before my postdoctoral thesis has more theoretical character. Therefore since I based my postdoctoral thesis on my father research activity, for long time the leader in research concerning breed improvement and reproduction in farm animals in Romania, I had to ask him to consent to publish a book and to be the first author. He considered that we can use more genuine results if we will limit the theme to the sheep species and I agreed. That explain why the theme is treated only in sheep and why is based mostly on provided research in Romania.

At the time I have started my PhD thesis plenty of reports concerning biotechnics of embryo transfer in dairy cattle had been published. Such reports referred to estrus synchronization, super ovulation, embryos recovery and preservation, transplantation of embryos to receptors. But few words existed about MOET. In an open discussion at the Veterinary Medicine Society of Romania M.Paraschivescu already presented "Hatchery Farm in Dairy Cattle Breeding" (1989)[2] a new idea of producing ET calves in closed farms, protected from disease contamination. About MOET in other species there was no word. Meanwhile, up to 2011 year when I started my postdoctoral training, some titles including "multiple ovulation" syntagma as for instance F.M.Bari's "Factors

---

[1] Paraschivescu, M.Th. *Studiu de proiect privind înființarea unei ferme MOET cu circuit deschis.* Teză de Doctorat, U.S.A.M.V.București, 2002
[2] Paraschivescu, M.; Mocanu, V.; Paraschivescu, Maria. *Hatchery Farm in Dairy Cattle Breeding.* Veterinary Medicine Society – Open discussions upon against diseases protection, 1989

affecting the survival of sheep embryos after transfer within a MOET program"[3] or "Multiple Ovulation and Embryo Transfer in Goats"[4] PhD thesis of Khoboso training, some titles affecting the survival of sheep embryos after transfer within a MOET program"[5] or "Multiple Ovulation and Embryo Transfer in Goats"[6] PhD thesis of Khoboso Christina Lehloenya have been published. Interesting knowledge concerning MOET in sheep and goats as practical tool for commercial activity is contented in Stela Zamfirescu and Al.Şonea's book "Reproduction Biotechnologies in Small Ruminants Breeding".[7] That means other research officers are interested in using MOET for the benefit of animal production as well. To think about virtues and servitudes of MOET in any fields of animal breeding became of current interest.

Now days the World is in under full demographic explosion. Food security and safety food are the major priorities of the animal sciences. Social division of labour led more and more to produce goods for market. Thus any business has to give profit in order to be sustainable. Farming makes no exception.

In principle the profit of sheep farm business equals the difference between the incomes obtained for the produced goods and the cost of outputs. Incomes primary depend of the price per unit of each kind of goods produced and secondary by the quantity of outputs. Price is established by market demand and it can't be controlled. The quantity of farm outputs can be increased by biotechnological means. Now days when virtues or servitudes of new methods in farming are discussed the question of profit is firstly implied.

Nevertheless the questions of food security and of safety food mustn't be neglected. Great attention is paid to the sustainable development and to the natural environment protection, as well. Future globalization of the World is expected. There are many reasons why spare outputs disclosed by reproduction biotechnologies in sheep and their virtues and servitudes can be considered undemonstrative.

Marcel Theodor Paraschivescu

---

[3] Bari, F.; Khalidb, M.; Haresign, W. *Factors affecting the survival of sheep embryos after transfer within a MOET program.* Theriogenology 59, 2003
[4] Khoboso, Christina Lehloenya. *Multiple Ovulation and Embryo Transfer in Goats.* PhD thesis, 2008
[5] Bari, F.; Khalidb, M.; Haresign, W. *Factors affecting the survival of sheep embryos after transfer within a MOET program.* Theriogenology 59, 2003
[6] Khoboso, Christina Lehloenya. *Multiple Ovulation and Embryo Transfer in Goats.* PhD thesis, 2008
[7] Zamfirescu Stela; Şonea Al. *Biotehnologii de Reproducere la Rumegătoarele Mici.* ISBN: 973-644-113-X

INTRODUCTION

Human population is increasing tremendously. We are now over 7 trillion of souls. The food security of the humankind is in danger. Energy crisis is a permanent menace. Protection of people health became a necessity. Every biological resource has to be economically used. Sustainable future existence of humanity is a main target for science and policy.

Sheep a before neglected farm animal species by countries with intensive agriculture have been studied less than cattle, pigs or poultries from the point of view of genesis (reproduction) function. So it disposes of appreciable reserves of fertility and productivity. These reserves must be disclosed.

The proposed theme of this book is to present authors' knowledge and opinion concerning reproduction and genomic biotechnologies in sheep and to assemble them in efficient farming systems that are using the current artificial biodiversity of this genetic species, in order to breed more valuable phenotypes of the desired type by breeders. The target assumed is rather difficult since sheep genetic species is spread all over the Earth, is kept mostly in close contact to the natural environment, disposes of sever molecular and behavioral mechanisms of closed reproduction and pertain to the sexual eukaryotic type of genetic information with a great number of gene loci and of allele genes per locus.

Perhaps sheep *(Ovis Arries)* was the first domesticated herbivorous species of mammals since the body weight of wounded or captured animals allowed *hunters* to move them in captivity and kept them as a reserve of food. Later when animals became able to reproduce in captivity the former hunters became *breeders* and got control over flocks' reproduction. They started to practice artificial selection by deciding which rams were allowed for mating and which offspring have to be slaughter and when. At the beginning breeders wanted to have mutton to eat and furs to cover their naked skin. Later they learned to eat sheep milk and discovered to use wool for tissues. Then they have isolated flocks of ewes with thin wool from flocks of ewes with thick wool and white ewes from black ewes and gave them rams of the same type. Afterward some milk was used for nurse children and part of it to prepare cheese. Finally breeders distinguished furs from pelts, distinguished fat mutton from lean mutton, and distinguished wool for carpets, with desired gross fibers, from wool for tissues (with desired thin or middle thin fiber) and from very thin wool with more expensive utilization.

Groups of sheep flocks have been reproductively insulated as specialized breeds for special productions.

A great artificial biodiversity of artificial populations has been created within the genetic species of *Ovis arries* while the natural, biological species *Ovis arries*, described by the old Taxonomy has disappeared. The diversity of goods produced with the sheep has created the great artificial biodiversity of sheep. Thus discussing general effects of reproduction biotechnologies in sheep is a mistake. Effects of biotechnologies have to be considered related to the goods produced by breeds and to the flock location on the Earth.

The theme isn't properly covered if biotechnological procedures are not entirely considered. Some authors include in biotechnologies al actions involving animals. Farming and even veterinary medicine are treated as biotechnologies. We don't agree. We think animal biotechnology must refer only to the genesis function or to bioengineering of one animal genetic species in course and its effects have to be discussed for each breed in case. That isn't an easy target but we will want to respect it.

This book is intended to be a synthesis of the question of virtues and servitudes of applying reproduction and genomic biotechnologies in sheep farming in the actual vision of the sustainable human society development, based on authors' results along their research activity. Therefore the authors, who are father and son, have cited in the text of the book plenty published titles by them in different circumstances. The first chapter of the book will be dedicated to the current biodiversity of sheep considering actual vision of the sustainable human society development concerning sheep industries as directory for the farming and science target. It is presented in a systemic way referring to the goals of breeding, systems of farming, types of products and sustainability. The second chapter will refer to reproduction (genesis function and breeding) in the genetic species of sheep. Other chapter is presenting knowledge about reproduction biotechnologies in sheep as resulted, mostly, of authors' scientifically research activity. The next chapter, what is a new minded one, intents to suggest how reproduction biotechnologies with sheep might help disclosing hidden resources for better productivity in different sheep farming systems.

Instead of conclusions some considerations about the most interesting opportunities of reproduction biotechnologies with sheep will be economically estimate having in mind the need for a sure gross margin of the farm economy, what means low variable costs, and how good gross profit could be when natural environment is used and protected as much as it is possible. Some considerations about the current main question of the World and how farm animal biotechnologies, as a whole, could be involved are emitted.

Chapter 1
THE GENETIC SPECIES OF SHEEP AND ITS BIODIVERSITY

Biological diversity concept

The beauty of the nature is given by its **biodiversity. Biodiversity** is result of the number of biological species. *A biological species (species* = kind of*) is the community of beings that reproduce among themselves (closed reproduction).*[8] Each biological species is support of one *species of genetic information.* The matter as reality around presents three forms of existence: *information,* as unity of *contraries,* **energy** as source of *movement* and **substance,** as the existence possessing *mass* (see *figure 1.1*).

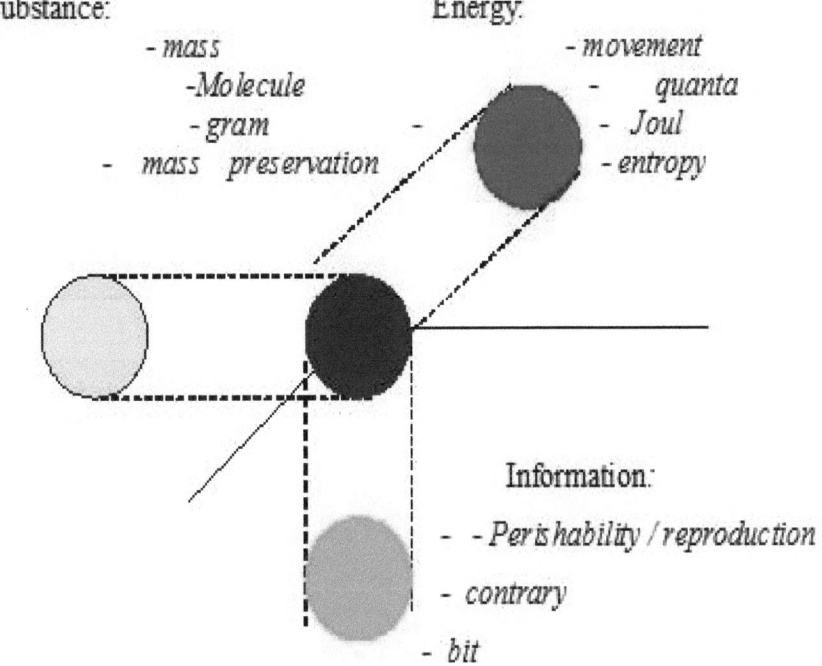

Fig.1.1. Matter unity: the three forms of its existence

---

[8] Paraschivescu, M. *Gnosis foundation of biological diversity.* Report at Rumanian Academy of Agriculture and Forestry Sciences, June 2011

The essential trait of information is *perishability with reproduction.* Information as anything else evolved[9] (see *fig.1.2).* There is ***fundamental information*** existing without support of energy or substance and there is ***information on support*** *of energy or substance.* There is also ***genetic information*** having as support *live substance* able of metabolism, organized as *biological spec*ies each of them being support for one *genetic species.* ***Species of genetic information*** and their live support, *biological species,* have been formatted in nature by *evolution under natural selection control,* as it was demonstrated by Charles Darwin.[10]

									Creative	
							Cognitive			
						Sensitive				
					Post-genetic Information					
				Eukaryote						
			Prokaryote							
			Genetic Information							
		Of substance								
	Of energy									
	Information on support									
Space										
Time										
Hazard										
Fundamental Information										

Fig.1.2. Evolving types of information

The biological species are formatted of individuals (organisms). In mammal animals species there are individuals of two sexes. When mature mammal *females produce ova* that are fertilized by mating, they become *pregnant, give birth to progeny* and *produce milk* to feed the new born progenies. *Male* animals *produce spermatozoa* and *mate females* to fertilize ova. Together *they ensure the reproduction of their **genetic species*** and the multiplication of species' individuals. The maintenance of genetic species and of their support is ensured by *natural mechanisms of closed reproduction,* genetically controlled by each kind of genetic species information. In mammals natural mechanism of closed reproduction are *molecular (Zona Pellucida reaction, the Vitellin block, the*

---

[9] Paraschivescu, M.; Paraschivescu, M.Th. *Psychic stress and animal welfare in dairy cattle production.* Scientific papers C series volumul LVIII (3), F.M.V.Bucureşti 2012, pag.194-203
[10] Mateescu, Raluca. *Marker Assisted Selection in Animal Breeding.* Training course at Animal Biology and Nutrition Institute, Bucharest, Romania, 2011

Karyotype, the Allele complementarities, the Major Histocompatibility Complex, the Maternal recognition of pregnancy)[11] and behavioral (*innate and conditioned nervous reflexes).*[12]
Individuals inside genetic species differ with their *sex* and present legitimate *variation of traits* induced by their genotypes *(variability).* The laws governing *the variability* of biological traits in case of closed reproduction are the *laws of chance,* the great discovery of Gregor Mendel.[13] Thus biological species have got the virtues of *populations of numbers* studied by *mathematical statistics.* Par consequence from the biodiversity point of view we must distinguish between *animal livestock* (number of heads) and *animal population* (the livestock resulted from closed reproduction). We have to conclude that in nature there are two kinds of biological diversity: *biodiversity* given by the biological species and *variability* given to individuals inside species when ova are fertilized by sperms inside of the biological process of reproduction (see the Convention for Biological Diversity – Rio de Janeiro (1992)[14] In fact we have to add the *biological diversity of cells* building up tissues, organs, apparatuses and physiologically systems.

Biodiversity in sheep

Now, concerning the genetic species of sheep, *Ovis arries,* mentioned in Taxonomy, no livestock of this kind is mentioned to exist as wild animals in nature. Old scientists thought domestic sheep derive from some biological species of wild ewes pertaining to genus *"Ovis".* Al.Furtunescu[15] repeating what former authors had written before says ancestors of domestic sheep are as follows: *Ovis musimon* (Muflon) have originated sheep with short tail. *Ovis orientalis arcar, Ovis arcar Nasonoff, Ovis arcar Exersman* and *Ovis vigneii arcar* (Arcar) are ancestors of sheep on long tail. Meanwhile *Ovis ammon* or *Ovis argali Pallas* (Argali) and *Ovis polei* (Cacigar) are ancestors of sheep with under skin depots of fat at hips or tail.

[11] Paraschivescu, M. *Molecular mechanisms of closed reproduction in mammal farm animals.* Simposium Iaşi, 2007
[12] Paraschivescu, M.Th.; Bogdan, A.T.; Paraschivescu, M.; Tobă, G.F.; Stan, Simona. *Biodiversity in farm animals: sources, using, conservation.* Lucrări ştiinţifice, Seria D vol.LII, U.S.A.M.V. Bucureşti 2009; pag.89-95
[13] Hartl, D.L.; Freifelder, D.; Snyder, L. *Basic Genetics.* Johnes and Bartlett Publishers Boston Portola Valley, 1988
[14] *Convention for biological biodiversity.* Rio de Janeiro, 1992
[15] Furtunescu, Al. *Zootehnie Generală.* vol.I, Editura Agrosilvică de Stat, Bucureşti, 1958

Recognition of so many biological species of the genus *Ovis* might be explained since the systemic classification of taxonomy is based on morphological traits of populations and such variability could be created by natural selection determined by territorial insulation of livestock. The question is if all these species enlisted by Taxonomy (some time with different names) are really genetic species. Deed they dispose of molecular mechanisms of closed reproduction? If they would dispose of such mechanisms the opinion that different breeds of domestic sheep originate from different wild genetic species is wrong since al crosses among domestic breeds result in fertile progeny. No genetically controlled mechanism of insulating reproduction was ever claimed. The answer to this question has importance in case of transferring genes in sheep genomes. We think more probable all present breeds of sheep originate from only one genetic information species, *Ovis arries,* that extinct in nature and prospered in culture losing its traits as biological population but keeping its natural mechanisms of closed reproduction. The actual high biodiversity of sheep genetic species is due to the accommodation of individuals to the biotopes of the large areal occupied by this species and to the diversification of artificial selection resulting from the evolution of humankind needs along times. Let's then classify the sheep genetic species biodiversity by its artificial biological populations, the breeds, not by ancestors.

From the point of view of when sheep breeds have been formatted it is possible to speck about ***native breeds, indigenous breeds, modern breeds*** and ***specialized breeds.***

Native breeds are the oldest ones. They resulted from the wild captured animals when people became *breeders,* what means they became able to feed and reproduce them. From ewes they were interested to have lambs and milk. From slaughtered animals they used mouton and furs. That time no improvement of production traits has been exercised. Nevertheless due to accommodation to hard natural conditions with two different periods one reach in feed and another poor in feed for sheep, a type disposing of "Kurdüc" (under skin depot of fat on tail or upper limb) was isolated in dry Central Asia and Mongolay. Now day native breeds are kept by nomad people where they still exist. Nomadic system is condemned to disappear and the native breeds as well. From the sheep biodiversity point of view the clever action is native breeds to be preserved at list *ex situ,* by freezing embryos, semen and tissues in order to preserve their genes.

Indigenous breeds have been created later, when human communities stopped migrating. They appeared especially after political boundaries led to formation of states were marked. One of the oldest breed in the South- East of Europe is the "Tzurcana" sheep, called also the "Valahian sheep". Valahia was the former name of the Romanian province located on the North river side of Danube. It is a light sheep able to walk long distances to feed and very resistant both to reins and dry weather. Also ewes of this breed are enough good milk producers. At present it is the main sheep population of Romania.

That time one of the traits of interest for humans has became the wool production. Populations of sheep with one type of wool fiber have been isolated. They were result of empirical artificial selection of genetic mutations. In the eastern part of Europe the "Tzigaia" type of sheep with the wool fiber diameter over 30 μ was isolated and the "Merino" type of sheep with the wool fiber diameter over 20 μ was isolated in South-east Asia. Tzigaia and Merino are indigenous types of sheep. Also indigenous breed is the Karakul breed developed in the central Asia for the beautiful pelts of new born lambs. It was formatted from "Kurdüc" sheep with fat tail.

Modern sheep breeds appeared in the eighteenth century when Robert Bakewell[16] practiced methodically artificial selection using one wanted type and one Flock Book as the mean to closed reproduction for each breed. The wanted type of the breed describes distinctly how rams must and how must ewes of the breed look and the least performances they have to express. The Flock Book is the artificial mechanism of closed reproduction giving the identity of the breed. It acts as a register enlisting the male and female genitors of the breed. The reproduction is closed since the no genitor is enlisted if both its parents hadn't been registered in the same Flock Book. Each genitor is enlisted with its identity. A nice definition of identity is given by one Romanian dictionary: *identity = similitude to itself.* That means identity has to include a name and a number (may be a code to) that individualize the genitor (even photo might be added if that help), data of its birthday, 2 or 3 generation of ancestors *(pedigree)* permitting to understand familiar relations, measured performances and important progeny. The genitors registered in the Flock Book must be marked, must receive markings attached to its body ensuring recognition of its individuality and identity. In old times markings were applied on the skin with hot up to red iron tools, or they were codified as notched and holes on the

---

[16] Mateescu, Raluca. *Marker Assisted Selection in Animal Breeding.* Training course at Animal Biology and Nutrition Institute, Bucharest, Romania, 2011

external ears. Not long after tattoos on the nude skin and ear tags have been applied noticing the register number. In the last time animals' identity includes the blood group or the DNA test if they were performed.

Bakewell who is considered as father of art of breeding is responsible for Shire horse, Leicester sheep and Long Horne cattle breeds.[17] Following the Bakewell's model many sheep breeds have been created in England: Leicester breed was appreciated for the body frame, for the length of wool fiber and for the fact that cross lambs from the Scottish Black Face, wanted in crossbreeding program for more mutton, have a gray face being easy to be recognized. Cheviot breed has good wool for tissues. The brown face Suffolk and the white face Romney Marsh have good mutton and Border Leicester disposes of the very interesting trait of a longer breeding season. There were more sheep breeds created in that time. What is for sure every breed can be recognized without mistake by its body type.

From the modern sheep breeds were developed the actual specialized breeds. The most famous are the Australian Merino for very thin wool, English Southdown for mutton, the Frisian sheep and the Israel's Awassy for milk yields, Karakul and one South Africa's sheep for pelts, Finish Landrace, Romanoff breed and Borula Merino have high prolificacy and so on. Some breeds whose production, as the milk or the mouton ones, require rich diets in energy and respond to the intensive farming. Production of thin wool or pelts can be obtained in the extensive farming. Light body weights are convenient in areas of poor feeding resources where animals have to walk long distances to satisfy their nourishment needs.

In addition to these remarkable biodiversity of the genetic species of sheep ingenious crossbreeding programs have been developed by breeders. Many such programs are applying reproduction biotechnologies.

Perhaps somebody will say all above information concerning Bakewell's way dealing with breeds are well known everywhere and there is no need to speak about. It isn't true. Much confusion exists concerning the correct meaning of the term "population" in animal breeding. Many authors are using the term "population" for the number of heads in a farm or in a district. From statistical point of view that is a mistake, a gross mistake, because trait inheritance laws of Mendel are ignored and unexpected results could be met.

---

[17] Pawson, H.C. *Robert Bakewell. Pioneer livestock breeder*. London : Crosby Lockwood & Son, Ltd, 1957

Population, in animal breeding, is a group of beings in closed reproduction (that reproduce inside the group). In statistics the simplest population of numbers is the one resulting out of $(a+b)^n$ relation controlled by the laws of chance. In nature biological populations are the biological species formatted by the laws of chance in closed reproduction controlled genetically by the species of genetic information commanding inheritance of traits. In culture the rule of closed reproduction has to be respected as well. Bakewell had succeeded in creating the Leicester breed because he had imagined the Leicester Flock Book and respected the use of it to close reproduction. He registered in the Leicester Flock book only lambs having both parents registered in the Leicester Flock Book.

It is true that from closed reproduction result similar organisms but that doesn't mean that all gray hair sheep are of the same breed. Other traits could differ. There are gray Tzurcana lambs and gray Karakul lambs, but the commercial quality of their pelts is not similar. During the planned economy of Romania many arbitrary rules were put to act instead of objective laws of the market or of the nature. Thus ignoring the efficiency of Bakewell's Flock Book and of closed reproduction in creating artificial farm animal populations, neglecting the Mendel's laws of traits inheritance and the importance of the wanted type of breeds many similar flocks were registered as breeds. Therefore the animal farm biodiversity has to suffer because the so called breeds, based only on some similitude of traits, weren't really artificial populations, but mathematically speaking them were mobs, with disordered variability, resulted from all kind of disjunctions induced by crosses. Since cross is considered in many other countries as method of breed improvement, one international convention in this respect would be useful. Crossbreeding doesn't create biodiversity in domestic sheep but destroys it. In fact cross breeding, which in nature doesn't act because of genetic species control of reproduction, in culture is the main cause of breeds' extinction. Most breeds extinct by crossbreeding when they lose their place as producers in the breeders' interest. Therefore we propose other grades of extinction risk for breeds than the one accepted by FAO after Rio de Janeiro convention for biological diversity.

We think that the 4 grades of extinction risk of mammalian species:
- Safe species having more than 10000 of adult females;
- Vulnerable species having 1000 – 10000 of adult females;
- Species in danger having 100 – 1000 of adult females;

- Species in critical state having less than 100 adult females, proposed by Rio de Janeiro are correct in wild life, because of natural mechanisms of closed reproduction controlled by genetic species.

But for the farm animal populations the same degrees of extinction risk proposed are wrong because they can lose their identity by crossing. Therefore we propose other classification that might be:

- Active breeds disposing of a Herd Book, Stud Book or Flock Book (related to the genetic species) and of proper breed improvement program;
- Breeds in safety, local native or indigenous breeds disposing of large number of females whose number of females remain nearly constant from year to year;
- Vulnerable breeds whose breeding stock is constantly decreasing from year to year, doesn't matter how many heads still exist in the breed;
- Breeds in danger whose breeding stock decreased under 1000 heads, pertaining to less than 6 families judged by three generation pedigrees;
- Breeds in critical state whose breeding stock has less than 100 heads pertaining to less than 4 families;
- Breeds in construction or reconstruction disposing of reproduction program and of a Flock Book for closed reproduction.

The breeds in safety would be really safe if they will become active breeds. Vulnerable breeds could be maintained if they are used in reasonable crossbreeding programs. The solution is recommended for the breeds in danger, as well. The breeds in critical states could be preserved *ex situ* as depots of embryos and semen. A better way is to reconstruct the breed up to the degree of a breed in danger and used it in reasonable crossbreeding programs. Working with sheep breeds in construction or in reconstruction requires using Flock Books, Wanted Type, one clear selection criterion (trait indicator or synthetic index) for reproductive discrimination and the necessary criteria to obtain the wanted type.

Identity in biological diversity of sheep

In working with farm populations of great importance is to individualize animals by marks in order to recognize their identity. Along the time method of marking animals in order to individualize their identity evolved. Perhaps the oldest one was notching the lobs of the external ears. In sheep ear notching is a very interesting procedure since it can't be lost or changed and can be used doesn't matter the ear color of lambs.

Later the deficiency of this procedure was considered that only small numbers could be marked. Herby we present a key for notching large numbers (see *figure 2* and *tables 1.1* and *1.2*). The innovation is using notches and holes to mark not numbers but exponents of number powers. The ear number is given by the sum of powers of numbers. In the example given number 2 is used as base of the power numbers.

Let us now to make some considerations concerning ear number of animals. As mean of individualization the ear numbers have the servitude of being more difficult to be memorized comparing to names, but they have the advantage to be more convenient for computing. At the same time ear numbers can offer more information about animals' identity than names. Long time ago, may be 50 years from now, in a brochure for beef cattle breeders we founded the idea of adding to the sign marked of animal skin in order to recognize property the last figure of the year when animal was born in order to know its age. Quite at the same time Fishteag I. acting as scientifically director of the Animal Science Research Institute of Romania disposed, for the Cattle Research Stations, to add behind the ear number of cattle, in horizontal position the last figure of the year of animals' birth. In 1967 when Paraschivescu M. conceived the register of artificial insemination points that were organized in Romania decided to use the last 2 figures of the animal's birth year in front of the ear number in order to have animals arranged with age adding new animals at the register end. For the species with shorter longevity than 10 years (sheep, pigs and poultry), he disposed only the last figure to be used. Next figures (one or two) might be used to indicate the animal family (of the father and of the mother).

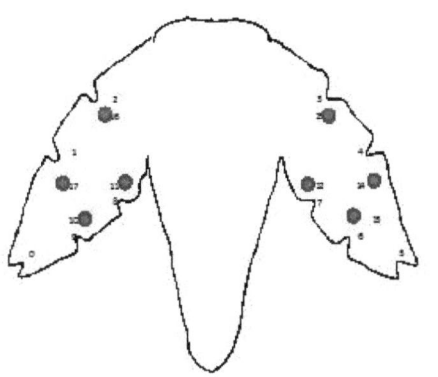

Fig.1.3. Key of exponent values (notches and holes)

The other part of the ear number, up to 7 figures in cattle, had to be given in order of birth, according odd numbers to males and even numbers to females.

The same rule was disposed for all other species using ear numbers of 6 or only 5 figures.

Let us suppose we want to mark the ear number of a male lamb of the family 5 and born by a mother of the family 3. He was born as the 98 lamb in 2009 year. Then the number must be 9, for the year of birth, 5 for his family (the same with his father family), and 3 for his mother family. Let us say he was the 95th born lamb supposing that up to his birth the number of ewe lambs was a little more than the number of ram lambs. Then for a number of 6 figures we will have to mark 953095. Now we have to find the power numbers in base 2 whose sum will give 953095.

Table 1.1.
Numbers responding to the power from 0 to 19 of the base number 2

0 - 4		5 - 9		10 - 14		15 - 19	
exponent	number	exponent	number	exponent	number	exponent	number
0	1	5	32	10	1024	15	32768
1	2	6	64	11	2048	16	65536
2	4	7	128	12	4096	17	131072
3	8	8	256	13	8192	18	262144
4	16	9	512	14	16384	19	524288

In order to find the component power numbers of the base number 2 we have to search the number with the most appropriate value to 953095 in table 1.1. This number is 524288 = 2^{19}. Then we must ad 953095 – 524288= 428807 to obtain the wanted ear number. The number whose value is most appropriate to 428807 is 262144= 2^{18}. Now we have to add 428807 – 262144 = 166663. The most appropriate value in the table is 131072 = 2^{17}. That means we need other 35591units what is 2^{15} + 2823. This time we have to use from the table the value 2048 = 2^{11} and will need other 775 units that we can obtain from 512 = 2^9+ 263. To have 263 we have to sum 256= 2^8+ 7. The number 7 is obtained from 4 = 2^2 + 3= 2^1 +1 = 2^0. It resulted that 953095 = 2^{19}+2^{18}+2^{17}+2^{15}+2^9+2^8+2^2 +2^1+2^0

That means we have to mark on the ear the holes for the exponents 19; 18; 17; and 15 and the notches for the exponents 9; 8; 2; 1; and 0.

For bigger numbers powers of base number 3 can be used (see table 1.2.).

Table 1.2.

Numbers responding to the power from 0 to 19 of the base number 3

0 - 4		5 - 9		10 - 14		15 - 19	
exponent	number	exponent	number	exponent	number	exponent	number
0	1	5	243	10	59049	15	14348907
1	3	6	729	11	177147	16	43046721
2	9	7	2187	12	531441	17	129140163
3	27	8	6561	13	1594323	18	387420489
4	81	9	19683	14	4782969	19	1162261467

Acting in the same manner as above us will find out that the wanted ear number will look like:

$$953095 = 3^{12}+3^{11}+3^{11}+3^{10}+3^8+3^6+ 3^6+3^5+3^3+3^2+3^2+3^1+3^0$$

That shows the resulted exponents that have to be marked. As it can be seen some exponents like 11; 6 and 2 are repeated what means two holes or two notches must be marked on the respective location.

The presented operation seems to be laborious. But it is so only for the first ear number. The next numbers are easy to format. One simple electronic calculator is of help.

Years after tattoo was used to mark register numbers. As number locations the inner side of the ear lobes or the skin of the axial zones is used.

The modern electronic marking is the best since the register number can't be modified and can to be read from distance.

The most interesting question to be answered in the future from the point of view of biodiversity is to have compatible breeds to intensive farming.

Chapter 2
PARTICULARITIES OF REPRODUCTION IN SHEEP

Reproduction seasonality

Sheep are mammals. Ewes give birth to live lambs and feed them with milk in the first 4 -5 weeks of their life. Milk secretion continues after lambs are wined if ewes are milked.

Lambing is seasonal. The old European manual explained the seasonal sexual activity in ewes as a consequence of dark and light balance within a 24 hours day, of the moderate temperature in the fall and of the better vegetation of herbs with the first rains of the autumn.

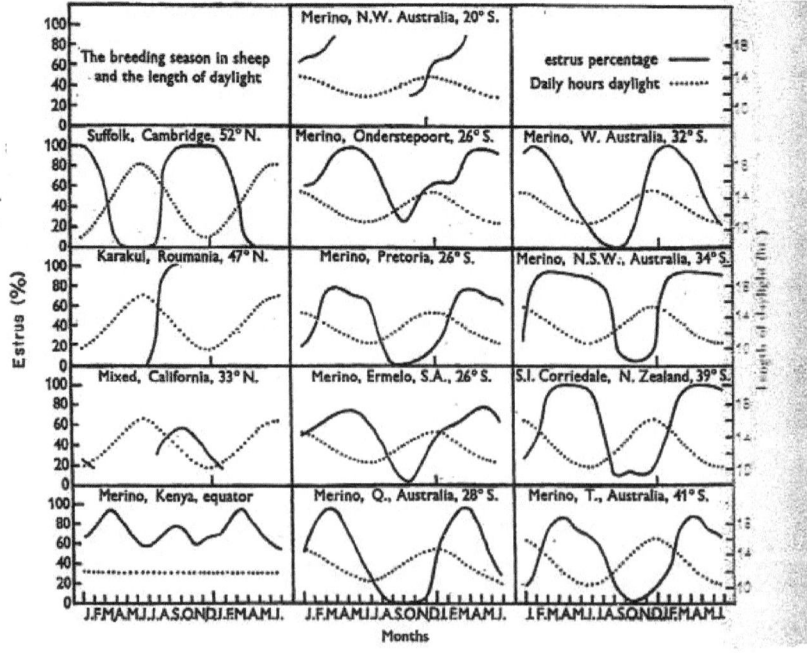

Fig.2.1. The relationship between the breading season and the length of daylight at different latitudes (Breed, locality and latitude are shown in that order in each graph.)
(From Hafez J.Agric.Sci., 42, 189)

Since these conditions are present in the spring as well, when ewes are lambing, now it is considered that the sexual activity is imposed in the fall trough natural selection by photoperiodism, by the diurnal periodicity of dark and light along the year time. The tendency of dark period increasing stimulates the optic centers and induces secretion of follicular stimulating hormone (FSH) by the pituitary gland and the secretion of the gonadotrophin realizing hormone (GnRH) by hypothalamus in ewes during the mating season when ewes show heats, accept mating, ovulate and are fertilized by rams' semen.[18] Sexual activity in rams follows the same pattern. Cumulated effect of the diurnal dark after the autumn equinox induces secretion of the testis interstitial cells stimulating hormone (ICSH) by the pituitary gland, what provokes testosterone secretion by testis and *libido* in rams.

The length of the mating season is controlled by photoperiodism and influenced by breeding systems. The graphics collected by Hafez are good arguments in this respect. See the continuous sexual activity of Merino sheep in Kenya, at equator, and the clear presence of anestrous in Suffolk sheep, at Cambridge at 52^0 north latitude.

Table 2.1.
Data concerning the mating season in S-E of Romania (44^0 latitude N)

Crt. no.	Farm code	Number of ewes	First day of estrus detection	Last day of estrus detection	% of first heat in the first 21 days	Last data with ewes in first heat	Period of first heat detection	Conception rate after the first artificial insemination
1	I	775	13.09	28.10	70,3	28.10	45	-
2	II	1448	15.09	02.11	79,0	1.11	47	-
3	III	1179	15.09	15.10	86,2	18.10	33	76,0
4	IV	1605	16.09	26.10	91,3	30.10	44	67,5
5	V	1051	21.09	12.11	100,0	12.10	21	-
6	VI	1223	21.09	11.11	86,8	27.10	36	-
7	VII	834	25.09	06.11	99,4	21.10	26	68,0
8	VIII	1331	01.10	08.11	92,4	8.11	39	95,0
9	IX	1271	01.10	11.11	88,2	9.11	40	-
10	X	534	01.10	09.11	87,8	9.11	40	69,0
11	XI	967	01.10	02.11	82,8	27.10	27	61,0
12	XII	855	01.10	11.11	88,2	7.11	38	-
13	XIII	764	01.10	12.11	88,5	1.11	32	62,0
14	XIV	884	01.10	08.11	98,7	24.10	24	71,5
15	XV	645	07.10	12.11	87,4	6.11	30	-
	Total	15366	13.09	12.11	x	9.11	57	

[18] Hafez, E.S.E. *Reproduction in Farm Animals*. Lea & Febiger, Philadelphia, 1962

The general rule is that at higher latitudes the anestrous period between two mating seasons is longer. The presented curves for Karakul in Romania (47^0 latitude N) and for Merino in NW Australia (20^0 latitude S) look differently because they don't show the distribution of ewes in heat during the mating season but the cumulated entrance of ewes in heat during the season. Nevertheless we have used sheep of Merionlandshaff breed bought from Germany having the breeding season in the spring.

The 15 points are part of a number of 96 points of artificial insemination with sheep where of 100566 breeding ewes received a first insemination, in the second year of PhD thesis of the first author of the present book.[19] The 15 points have been chosen as presenting the best registration of data and to cover almost the interval of dispatching semen from the artificial insemination center.

In *Figure 2.2.* the curve of daily estrus detection is presented. The sheep farms are enlisted in the order of beginning artificial insemination. The first farm opens its activity at September 13 and the last one in October 7. The peak of the curve was registered at October 1 and is due to management measures. It could be considered that intensive sexual activity in ewes is present after 21 of September. The farm what registered 100% of first insemination in its flock had animals in good body condition. The length of sexual season is 3 times longer or more than the medium length of the estrus cycle (17 days) in ewes.

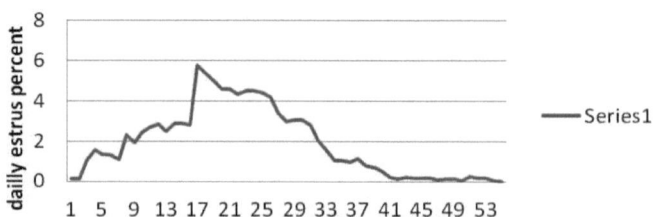

Fig.2.2. Mating season in ewes (440 N latitude) starting with 15th of September

Ewes in estrus means ewes accepting to be mated by rams, or to express the so called *"immobility syndrome"*. Estrus or heat lasts 36 hours as a mean in sheep. Sexual behavior of ewes is relatively inconspicuous and is not evident in the

[19] Paraschivescu, M. *Contribuții la cunoașterea și îmbunătățirea procesului tehnologic din centrele mari de însămânțări artificiale la oi.* PhD Thesis, Veterinary Medicine Faculty, Bucharest, Romania, 1963

absence of the ram.[20] Even the ewe in heat seeks out for the ram the only real evidence of estrus is the immobility syndrome, the willingness of ewe to allow the ram to tease her and mount. More difficulty of heat detection is added by the low height of sheep and by the large number of ewes in flock. The data above have been got using aproned teaser rams. It was denied using vasectomized teaser rams in order to prevent spreading of *Brucella ovis* (*varietas australiae*) infection in flocks. The *Brucella ovis* infection is causing epididymitis and sterilization of rams but no abortion in ewes. The measure was important since in all the flocks free mating was provided to fertilize ewes returning in heat after artificial insemination ceased. The percentage of unfertilized ewes after artificial insemination might be estimated to vary between 10% to 15% or more.

Estimation of conception rate was done by the *fast non return rate* procedure as we called it. The *fast non return rate* is a genuine procedure that compares the total number of repeated heats after insemination with the total ewes' number reported as artificially inseminated 17 days before the day of the estimation, up to.

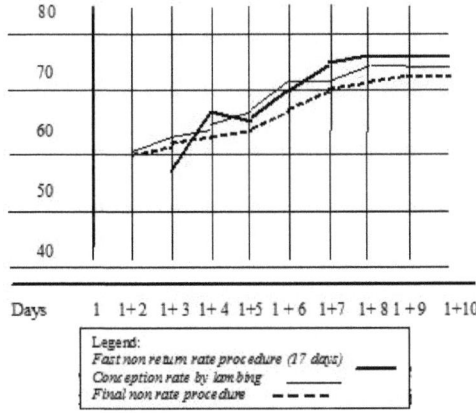

Fig.2.3. Estimation of conception rate in artificially inseminated ewes

The precision of fast non-return rate procedure *(Fig.2.3)*[21] was demonstrated with the data in a flock of 506 artificially inseminated ewes. Therefore conception rate estimation *counting* the quotient of total number of ewes that returned in heat up to the day of counting with *the number of inseminations*

[20] Paraschivescu, M. *Reproducția la Ovine,* Editura Agrosilvica, 1969
[21] idem

performed up to 17 days before the day of counting (the fast non return rate conception) has been compared to the quotient of fertilization estimated by the *final non return rate* in the flock and the quotient of conception rate counted by registered parturitions. Parturitions are giving the most precise information about the obtained fertility but information is very late, six month after mating season is closed. The final non return conception rate estimation can be done in the autumn but after heat detection is finished. The fast non return rate estimation of fertilization gives the advantage of deciding the term at which AI can be stopped. The procedure can start with the first day of ewes returning in heat and became credible 3 days later. After other 3 days it becomes sufficiently sure for a correct estimation of artificially insemination's result. That gives the possibility to decide when the desired quota of fertilized ewes out of artificial insemination is attained and the rams might be introduced in flock for natural mating.

Puberty age in sheep differs with the farming system and with the breed. Lambs of native and local breeds fed extensively on natural pastures show heat or libido in the autumn of the second year of life, what means at the about 18 months of age. Lambs of improved breeds for mutton became able for reproduction after 6 months of age, in their first year of life. In this respect the energy concentration of diets and the farming system are decisive. Nevertheless there is some genetic control of the ability for feed consumption and of the feed conversion potential. The shepherds know very well what is better for their flocks.

Lambing interval and the fertility in sheep

Structure of the lambing interval is presented in *Fig.2.4.* Generally speaking the length of the interval between two successive parturitions is one year. It is determined by photoperiodism and/or by vegetation stages of herbs induced by climate.

After event of parturition ewes are suckling lambs. How long lambs suck differ very much. To get pellets lambs are slaughtered in the first 3 days of life. Lambs for Easter weighting 10 – 15 kg and of about 4 - 6 wicks of age are required in South-east of Europe. Two tooth lambs of 30 – 35 kg are preferred in the UK and in countries of English culture influence. In Mongolay lambs are slaughtered in the second year of live in order to be able to format tallow depots containing vitamins.

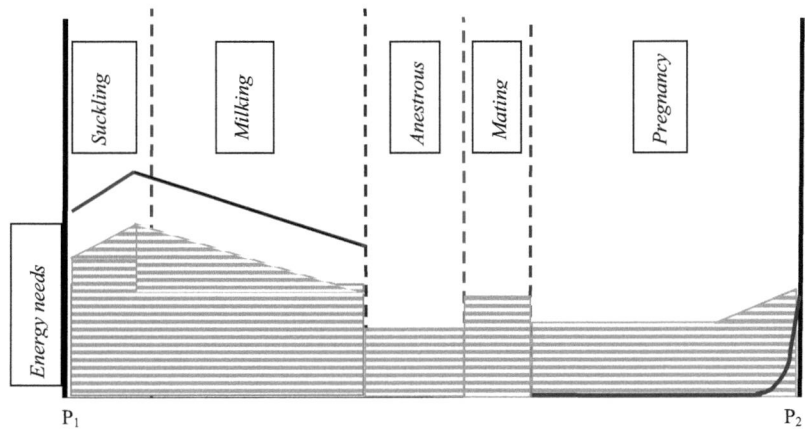

Fig.2.4. Structure of lambing interval

The presence of lambs induces anestrous through the optic centers action and hypothalamus on the pituitary gland. In farms where lambs are slaughtered early and the cost of labor is low, ewes are milked. There are also specialized breeds for milk production as the mentioned before the Friesian and the Awassy breeds. The harvested milk yield depends of the milked daily yields and of how long ewes are in milk. The first trait is improved by grading up selection of sheep populations; the second one has to be controlled by management. Anestrous persists after winning of lambs or after let of milking and the estrus cycles will appear as effect of photoperiodism, yet by artificial insemination without any medical treatment was possible to obtain lambing before the New Year. Earlier lambing became possible only step by step wining one gametogenic cycle of the ovary (17 days) in successive years. Of course genetics is implicated as well being much difficult to shift the sexual season in native breeds.

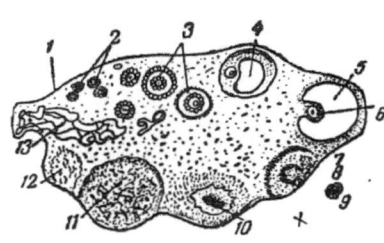

Fig.2.5. Ewe's ovary
1-germinal epithelium; 2- primary
follicles; 3- maturing follicles;
4- de Graaf follicle; 5.- ovulation;
6-ovocyt ; 7-opened follicle;
8-coagulated blood; 9-expulsed ovum;
10-young yellow body; 11 mature yellow
body;12- corpus albicans; 13-blood vessel

The mating is a complex act especially from the female part. In order to be mated the ewe has to accept the mount of the ram. That happens when she is in heat, when antral ovarian follicles secret estrogens inducing the sexual desire and one or two ovarian follicles break out (ovulate) to liberate ova that might be fertilized. All these things take place in ovarian cycles *(Fig.2.5)*.[22] Each ovary cycle has two phases one induced by estrogen hormones secreted by ovarian follicles and one induced by progestagen hormones secreted by *"corpus lutei"* (yellow bodies) formatted at the place of the broken off follicles. The two ovary cycle phases are called the follicular phase and respectively the luteal phase. The follicular phase is induced apart from equator areas by the shortening of the daylight period. This stimulus is transmitted to optic centers and from there to hypothalamus and to the pituitary gland which secretes the follicular stimulating hormone (FSH) commanding the growth of follicles up to the stage of dehiscent follicle (de Graaf follicle) and the luteinizing hormone commanding follicle dehiscence and the yellow body formation. The two mentioned gonadotrophins are released from the pituitary gland by the same hypothalamic hormone called Gonadotrophin Releasing Hormone (GnRH). GnRH currently releases any time the gonadotrophic hormones pituitary gland produces at that moment. FSH commands a wave of primary follicles to grow by multiplication of the granulose cells around the ovum and builds up an antrum that accumulates follicular liquid, surrounded by two peripheral thecae. The external theca nurses the follicle. The internal peripheral theca of the antral follicles acts as the gland secreting estrogen hormones. Estrogen hormones accumulate in the follicular liquid and at the climax induce the sexual desire of ewes. No new follicle is generated by the FSH action. The ovum in the primary follicle stays in the meiotic arrest of the firs meiotic division of ovocyte that had taken place during the embryonic stage of ontogenesis. This way the singularity and the stability of genetic information species are preserved.

Reproduction Systems

Reproduction systems could be genealogically classified as free and controlled. Free mating comports to leave free more rams in a flock along the entire mating season. Usually the target for a ram is 30 – 50 ewes. That is the oldest reproduction system of sheep breeding. It is practiced in extensive farming, is cheap and ensures the best fertility of the flocks. Servitudes of the system are the lack of protection against venereal diseases and a very slow flow of genetic

---

[22] Paraschivescu, M. *Reproducția la Ovine,* Editura Agrosilvica, 1969

progress. Controlled genealogy is possible using natural mating or artificial insemination. There are two controlled reproduction systems based on natural mating. One of them which we will call *restricted natural mating* implicates detection of ewes in heat by approved teaser ram and encloses the ewe in heat in the pen of the nominated ram for 3 days to be mated. This system is used in research trials since it permits a correct and detailed registration of data but it ask much labor and is costly. The second one, that we will call *harem mating,* is successfully applied on large scale in New Zeeland. In a large paddock a ram receive the ewes he has to mate and they stay together up to the lamb harvest and a new mating season. The system is sure and cheap. The only one care is to ensure a good insulation of *harems.* A very interesting *harem mating* is practiced by countrymen in a narrow area of Romania, nearby the Danube River, breeders of *"Karabasha"* sheep breed. The name "Karabasha" is not Romanian. It is formatted of two, may be Turkish, words: "Kara" that means *black* and "Bash" what means chef or *head.* As the name of the breed suggest it was brought from Asia but when and how we don't know. Animals of the breed are large, up to 90 – 100 kg live body weight in females and the daily milk yield over 2 kg per day, in the first part of lactation. Each husbandry of countryman families disposes of one *sheep harem* made up from 70 ewes and 1 ram. The interesting thing is that the ram is introduced in the flock as a yearling and is kept up to the oldest possible age. That means the ram will mate his daughters, his nephews and even his grand nephews in a close inbreeding what gives a high uniformity of the flock. But when the ram is called off because of the age, the new ram is taken from other husbandry usually from other village. Thus Karabasha breeders use inbreeding for increased homozygosis, avoiding at the same time concentration of lethal genes in the population. Artificial insemination with sheep presents servitudes connected with the needed labor, the difficulties of depicting ewes in heat and the quota of semen doses used for insemination in case of short term semen preservation. There are less difficulties concerning reproduction seasonality in rams. Conditioned reflexes of reproduction can develop libido without hormonal treatment.

Pregnancy is the final target of reproduction. Length of pregnancy in sheep is about 150 days. There is a variance due to the sex of the fetus, to the weight of the fetus, to the number of fetuses, and of course to the breed. Number of fetuses varies with the breed and the level of feeding in the mating period. Uterus sustains the pregnancy nursing fetuses' trough placenta. At the same time placenta acts as barrier that impedes infections to pas from mother to developing embryos. After parturition the free of content or pus uterus can secret $F_{2\alpha}$ prostaglandin ($PgF_{2\alpha}$). It has been demonstrated $PgF_{2\alpha}$ causes lysis of the yellow bodies that have sustained the pregnancy and induces uterus involution giving way to a new ovarian ciclicity, in cow. $PgF_{2\alpha}$ causes lysis of the yellow bodies in ewes, as well. Recent research has found out existence of the maternal recognition of pregnancy, one of the natural mechanisms of closed reproduction that preserves the purity of genetic species when they reproduce themselves.

Ram lambs get puberty in the second year of life at about 16 – 18 months of age in most breeds. In mutton breeds puberty is expressed in the first year of life at 5-7 months of age. Rams are lesser sensible to photoperiodism. Conditioned reflexes permit to obtain libido by training without any hormonal treatment. The individual volume of ram ejaculates varies between 0,5 and 1,8 ml. In one our research from 33 rams of Merino type, a total number of 1729 ejaculates were collected with a medium of 1.1 ml. The largest volume of one good ejaculate measured 3.8ml. Individually, per ram, the lowest mean volume measured 0,6 ml and the highest one measured 1,8 ml. In other experiment from 112 young rams, also of Merino type, 3804 ejaculates were collected. This time the mean value of ejaculates was 0,8 ml. The minimum mean in one ram was 0,5 ml and the maximum mean per ram was 3,8 ml. Ram semen has high density. Concentration of spermatozoa in normal ejaculates is 4 – 5 trillions per ml and more than 89% of sperms are motile.

Parturition is easy. Dystocia or placenta retention is very rear. Very few cases of metritis are reported. May be some cases recover during the long anestrous period from lambing to mating. Nevertheless cases of fetid pus were found when progestagen pessaries to block the ovary cycle have been extracted.[23]

General fertility in sheep genetic species disposes of hidden resources related to the structure of the lambing interval and the frequency of polyovulation and lambing of twins.

---

[23] Paraschivescu, M..; Ursescu, Al. *Sincronizarea estrului la ovine III. Frecvenţa stărilor anestrale.* Revista de Zootehnie şi Medicină Veterinară nr.10, 1968

Chapter 3
BIOTECHNOLOGICAL PROCEDURES IN SHEEP REPRODUCTION

Reproduction biotechnologies include any procedure intended to increase individual fertility in animals over the limits determined by the genetic species information of population. There are biotechnologies addressed to the male side or to the female side of the reproduction process and biotechnologies addressed to the genomic structures of reproduction.

Reproduction biotechnologies concerning the male side

Biotechnologies concerning the **male side** of reproduction resulted in the complex biotechnology of *artificial insemination.* The main components of artificial insemination are: *semen collection, semen dilution and partition in insemination doses, short term or long term preservation of semen, dispatching of insemination doses to flocks, detection of ewes in heat, inoculation of seminal material and estimation of conception rate.*

Semen collection with artificial vagina is perfect. Electro ejaculator use causes stress and requires too much labor. Some problems could be met in teaching rams of lymphatic or phlegmatic nervous type to artificial vagina. These rams require more attempts up to success collection and in the phlegmatic type inhibitor factors as for instance a too warm vagina could cause further refuse of the mount. Good disinfection of artificial vaginas has to be provided in order to prevent venereal diseases diffusion. Infectious epidimitys caused by Brucella Ovis varietas Australia is transmitted by natural mating and by non disinfected artificial vagina as well.

Semen dilution acts in two directions. It helps preserving sperms viability for longer time and permits ejaculate partition in feasible insemination doses. For short time conservation of semen dilution is done in synthetic medium containing 20% egg yolk, glucose and sodium citrate. One ejaculate having a volume of 1,2 ml and a concentration of 4 billion sperms per 1 ml contains 48'000'000'000 spermatozoa what are inseminated with 1 natural mating. For fertilization of the expulsed ova 20'000'000 live sperms are enough. If the ejaculate is not diluted this number of spermatozoa are contained in a volume of 0,005 ml, too small of a volume to be easy manipulated. If the semen is diluted 1/10 the volume of a dose becomes 0,05 ml what is a reasonable size. Usually

1/7 dilution is used for ejaculates whose volume measures 1 – 1,8 ml and 1/12 dilution is used for bigger ejaculate if sperms' concentration isn't decreased. The reason of this dilution degree is that at the primary dilution the volume of added medium is equal with the volume of the ejaculate and at the final dilution other 5 or respectively 10 times the ejaculate's volume of synthetic medium is added. Sometimes the preferred volume of insemination dose is 0,1 ml much easier to be measured. Then the degree of dilution can be increased. Fresh diluted semen is packed in 10 ml phials or in small pots of 10 ml. Of course in a pot is placed the diluted semen resulting from on ejaculate. Deep frozen semen is prepared as small pelts or in mini straws.

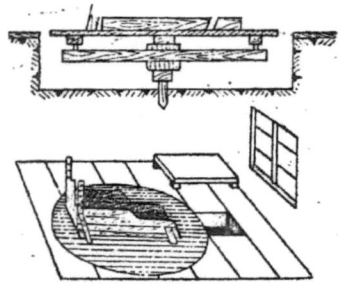

Fig.3.1.–Single place rotating stand for inseminating ewes

Semen inoculation must be done to ewes that are in heat only. Since estrus is 36 hour long the insemination is repeated after 24 hours. Insemination of ewes takes place in the morning after ewes in heat have been depicted. One dose of seminal material, diluted semen, is inoculated in the cervix. That could be done using a tubular vagina speculum and a frontal lamp. Insemination is repeated next day before stating the heat detection of the day. For more commodity of the inseminator a fixed or better a rotating stand at the floor level is recommended.

Detecting of ewes in heat is a laborious work limiting interest for current use of artificial insemination. In ewes heat is not evident in absence of ram and teaser rams have to be used. Aproned teaser rams, what means rams equipped with an apron covering ram's penis, left free among ewes is the best mean of heat detection. Other procedures like use of vasectomized rams or of rams with surgically deviated penis are less convenient since it is more costly and in case of vasectomized rams excludes the prophylactic advantage of artificial insemination. Only aproned rams could afterwards artificial insemination be used for the saving natural mating. Data presented in *table 2.1* from the previous chapter show that quota of unfertilized ewes had varied between 5% and 39%.

Dispatching semen to farms confronts with plenty of questions. In case of short term preservation of semen with daily expedition of it synchronizing the number of insemination doses send to flocks to the number of ewe in heat is impossible. If the fresh or the refrigerate semen is preserved for two or three days less doses of semen are lost. A problem is getting semen to isolated far located flocks. We have used small plains. Of cause copters are better. But there are 2 ways to reduce cost and losing semen, blind insemination after estrus synchronization in ewes or long term preservation of semen by freezing. The first way is cheaper and fertilization rate is higher.

Conservation of semen seems to be important. Collected semen is perishable. It can't be sent from artificial insemination centre to flock farms. Semen must be refrigerated or frozen.

Short term preservation can be obtained by refrigeration with ice under egg yolk protection. That is a satisfactory method from the point of view of fertilization results, but dispatching semen every day or even every two days is very costly. For semen transport refrigerators and cars are used. We had god results dispatching doses of semen by plan. Service small plane equipped with one refrigerator box received the doses of semen packed in small glass pots for each insemination point. The pots were thrown from plane from a low altitude attached to a simple paper parachute at a known point. This way flocks located far of accessible road were served.

Long term conservation of seminal material was obtained by freezing. First success we have got using dry ice (solid CO_2) for fast freezing small pellets of semen. Later liquid Nitrogen was used to freeze semen in thin straws. Poor hygiene at ewe flock locations, the needed equipment to thaw the frozen straws, the cost of cryogenic equipment and the seasonality of reproduction are reason why using frozen semen for artificial insemination didn't spread in sheep. Freezing semen for breeds' *ex situ* preservation seems to be nevertheless justified.

Biotechnologies concerning the female side

Biotechnologies concerning the **female side** refer to *estrus synchronization* and to *multiple ovulation embryo transfer (MOET)*.

Estrus synchronization appeared as a necessity of synchronizing the day of ovarian cycle of receptors with the age of embryo in case of embryo transfer. Lamond,[24] one of the first scientists working in this field, explained that in fact estrus synchronization means to induce estrus at the wanted moment, and that is true. There are two ways us to shift the ovaries' cycle. One way is to **block the**

---

[24] Lamond, D.R. *Animal Breeding Abstract*. 32 p., No.3, 1964

ovarian cycle in diestrus using progestagen hormones; the second one is to **interrupt diestrus by yellow bodies' lisis**.

First experiment[25] concerning estrus synchronization in ewes using progesterone was based on literature information. It was organized on local Merino sheep in the month of October. Synthetic results of the experiment are presented in table 3.1. Results have shown 29 days term for all flock the control lot to come in heat, and shorting this term to 8 days in the best experiment variant and to 19 days in the worst one. This difference in the experimental lots was due to the timing of progesterone administration. Worse result, quite no one, was obtained when a triple dose of progesterone has been given at three days interval. The 2 days interval between progesterone injections was not acceptable, too.

Table 3.1.
Estrus synchronization in ewes by blocking ovarian cycle with progesterone

Lots	Number of heads	Progesterone treatment			FSH treatment dose	Days with ewes in heat		Fertility (%)	
		Doze per treatment	Treatment interval	Number of treatments		Order number	Total number	After first cycle	Final fertility
I	50	20 mg	48 hours	7	-	1 – 13	13	86,0	100,0
II	50	20 mg	48 hours	7	800 IU	3 – 10	8	84,0	87,5
III	50	30 mg	72 hours	3	-	1 - 13	13	34,5	97,0
IV	50	30 mg	72 hours	3	800 IU	3 - 16	14	64,0	88,9
Control	50	-	-	-	-	1 - 28	28	96,0	96,0

Since results weren't satisfactory some questions arouse. Weren't part of ewes still in anestrous since in the control lot 29 days had been necessary for ewes to show the first heat? Was it correct to use dose of 10 mg progesterone per day and per ewe at two days interval but not daily? The term of 13 days when progesterone was inoculated was it long enough?

In order to answer these questions a trial to establish the minimal active dose able to maintain the diestrus state of the ewe has been done. This experiment[26] used 100 ewes of one research station located at the latitude about 44^0 N. Detecting the ewes in heat, using 5 aproned teaser rams, started in 18 of

---

[25] Oţel, V.; Harshianu, A.; Paraschivescu, M. *Sincronizarea estrului la ovine I.* Lucrări ştiinţifice ale ICZ vol. XXIV, Bucureşti, 1966
[26] Paraschivescu, M.; Ursescu, A.; Lepădatu, C. *Sincronizarea estrului la ovine III.* Revista de Zootehnie şi Medicină Veterinară, nr.12, Consiliul Superior al Agriculturii, 1968

September. In order to be sure that the flock had enter in the sexual season for 4 days no treatment was done. The sum of ewes in heat was 20 % of the flock livestock and ewes in heat were detected every day. Then we started daily administration of progesterone with the dose of 2 mg per ewe and increasing further the dose with 1 mg per day. So after 2 days since the percent of ewes in heat was similar to the one of the previous days the dose of progesterone was increased to 3 mg. for the next 2 days. We further increased every 2 days the progesterone dose. When the daily progesterone dose got to 10 mg no ewe in heat was more detected in the next 4 days. The experiment has given us a precise answer. Since 96 % of ewes enter in heat in the 18 days of heat detection it was clear that in full sexual season the daily dose of progesterone able to block the ovarian cycle is 10 mg. (see *Fig. 3.2).*

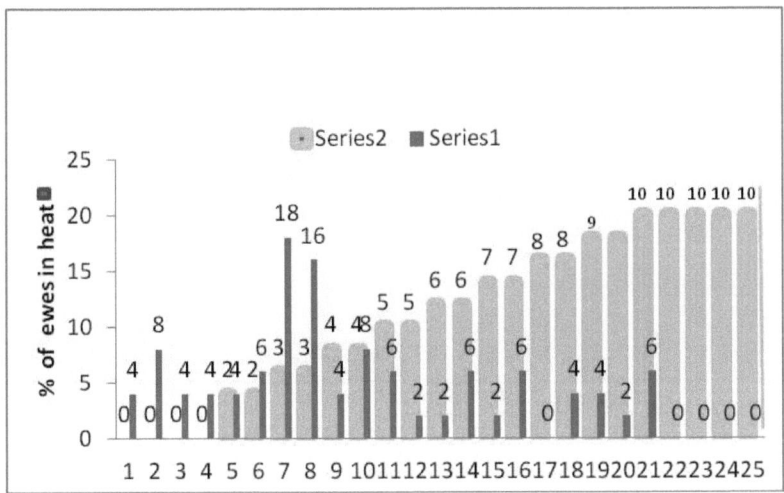

Fig.3.2. Minimum active doze of progesterone

It remained to answer the question about what long the term of progesterone treatment must be and if this term could be shortened by using gonadotrophin.

On this purpose the third experiment was organized.[27] This time experiment started in September 2 with 100 ewes which were distributed in five lots of 20 heads. Registered data are shown in *Fig.3.3.* and in *Table 3.1.*

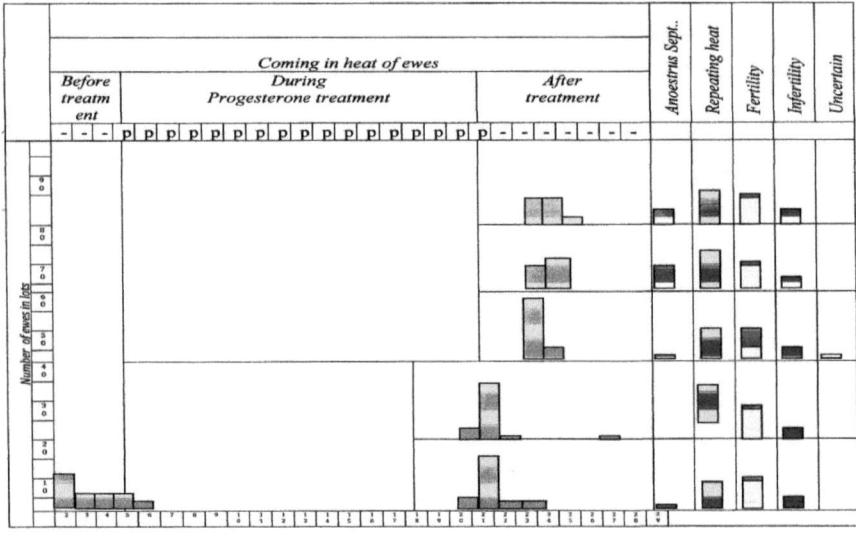

Fig.3.3. - Results of estrus synchronization – third experiment

As it can be seen from *Table 3.1.* and from the graphic in *Fig.3.3.* two lots (A_1 and A_2) received 10 mg progesterone daily for 13 days and 3 lots (B_1, B_2 and C) received progesterone for 16 days. On the other hand two lots of ewes (A_1 and B_1) received serum gonadotrophin (Roussel) and other two lots (A_2 and B_2) received Prolan A (Bayer). One lot of ewes (C) that received progesterone for 16 days didn't receive gonadotrophin. For detecting ewes in heat aproned teaser rams were used. Ewes in heat have been inseminated with fresh refrigerated semen prepared in the previous day. Detection of ewes in heat was continued and returned ewes were inseminated. At the end of experiment all ewes were put together in one flock and 5 rams were included for free natural mating. In the spring lambing was registered and results of inseminations and natural mating were estimated. The term of 16 days for the progesterone treatment was inspired by the fact that in the previous experiment the first ewes in heat were registered

---

[27] Oţel, V.; Paraschivescu, M.; Petria, I. *Sincronizarea estrului la ovine II.* Lucrări ştiinţifice ale ICZ vol.XXV, 1967

48 hours after the last progesterone injection denoting a 1 day length of proestrus.

Best estrus synchronization in ewes by progesterone intramuscular injection was obtained using daily doses of 10 mg for 16 days.[28] Association of Gonadotrophin to the last progesterone injection concentrates heat in 2 days interval but a big number of ewes receiving progesterone for 16 days didn't show heat after treatment. Since adding 800 IU of serum gonadotrophin (Roussel) increased the incidence of lambing twins, there is chance to increase ewes fertility if such treatment is applied at the start of proestrus to inducing follicular stimulation in the next ovarian cycle.

There were many ewes that returned in heat after the first artificial insemination. Return in heat has taken place after approximately one estrus cycle. This time heat has been synchronized on a bit longer term of about 5-6 days. These ewes were inseminated for the second time. In order to save the final fertility of the experimental lots then one single flock was formatted and 5 rams was allowed for free mating. Nevertheless in each lot 15% or 20 % of ewes were infertile since didn't give birth to lamb.

Since it was suspected that the registered infertility was due to many cases of anestrous in the time of natural mating next year a forth experiment to understand if progesterone treatment causes or doesn't cause anestrous was organized. In this experiment 3 lots were used one control lot with untreated eves, one experimental lot where ewes received daily 10 mg progesterone parenteral injection for 16 days and a second experimental lot receiving in addition to the last progesterone injection 800 IU of serum gonadotrophin (Roussel).[29] Results concerning estrus synchronization are presented in *Fig.3.4.* Results concerning anestrous incidence are presented in *Table 3.2.*

---

[28] Paraschivescu, M.; Ursescu, Al. *Sincronizarea estrului la ovine IV. Durata progesteronemiei induse și efectul gonadotrofinelor.* Revista de Zootehnie și Medicină Veterinară, nr.11, 1969
[29] Paraschivescu, M.; Ursescu, Al. *Sincronizarea estrului la ovine V. Frecvența stărilor anestrale.* Revista de Zootehnie și Medicină Veterinară nr.10, 1970

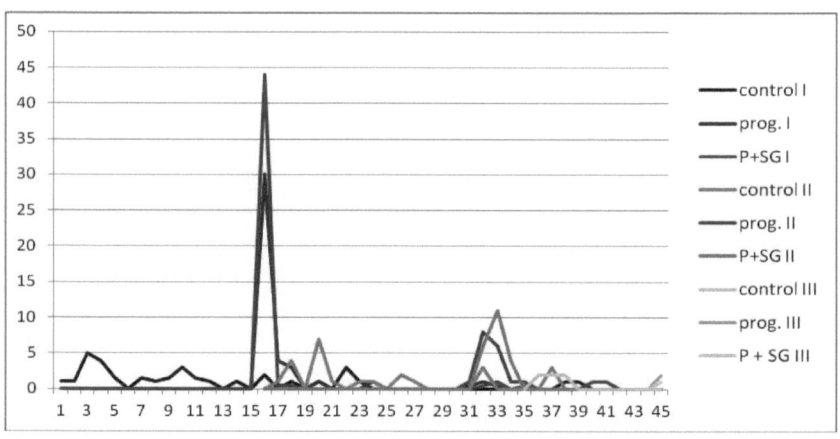

Fig.3.4. Estrus synchronization using progesterone injections

Table 3.2.

Data of the third experiment concerning estrus synchronization by blocking ovarian cycle

Lot	Treatment (10mg progesterone + gonadotrophin at the last progesterone injection)	Heads	Time from last progesterone dose to first heat (hours)				Return in heat cases		Lambing from the first insemination			Total lambing	Infertility	Unknown state
			48	72	96	120	Total in heat	Sept.	Oct.	Single	Twins.			
A₁	13 days progesterone + Gonadotrophin Roussel	20	3	14	2	2*	20	-	7	8	1	16	4	-
A₂	13 days progesterone + Prolan A 400 IU	20	3	15	1	-	19	1	10	6	1	17	3	-
B₁	16 days progesterone + Gonadotrophin Roussel	20	16	3	-	-	19	-	8	3	5	17	3	1***
B₂	16 days progesterone + Prolan A 400 IU	20	6	8	-	-	14	-	10	6	1	17	3	-
B₃	16 days progesterone	20	7	7	2	-	16	-	9	7	1	17	3**	-

* ewes that presented heat 2 days before;

** one ewe was in heat in October;

*** lost of the ear mark

In the control lot of 43 ewes' 38 ewes enter in heat during 24 days. Other 2 ewes were depicted 16 days later (probably undiscovered by teaser rams in the first cycle). In the first experimental lot 30 ewes enter heat in 3 days (20 of them in the 16th day, 6 in the 17th and 4 in the 18th day of heat detection) and other 2 ewes two days later. A number of other 6 ewes were detected in heat in three successive days at 15 days from the peak day of the former ovarian cycle (should be they weren't discovered by rams? It might be possible.).

Adding 800 IU of SG (Roussel) it improved estrus synchronization of ewes. At 48 hours from the last progesterone injection and in same day as in the experimental lot I, 27 ewes enter heat and other 4 ewes enter heat in the next 2 days. That means 86, 11% of ewes enter heat in 3 days. The rest of 5 ewes were detected in heat during 4 days sixteen days later (again suspicion that they were in heat 17 days before).

Concerning the incidence of anestrous and infertility cases as final results in the three lots of ewes there were little differences (*Table 3.3*). As anestrous cases ewes that weren't discovered in heat for the first, second or third insemination has been considered. Final anestrous was declared in ewes that showed no heat and didn't give birth to any lamb. As infertile ewes the ones that were once or more in heat but didn't conceive have been considered.

Table 3.3.

Results of the forth experiment for estrus synchronization in ewes

Experimental lot	Estrus cycle	Ewes%	Anestrous		Insemination		Parturition		Infertility	
			No.	%	No.	%	No.	%	No.	%
Control 43 ewes	I	43	3	69,77	40*	93,02	10	23,26	30	75
	II	33	9	13,95	24	55,81	8	33,33	16	23,26
	III	25	19	13,95	6	6,98	2	33,33	4	4,65
	mating	23	x	x	x	x	8	34,78	15	65,22
	Final	**43**	**1**	**2,33**	**70**	**162,79**	**28**	**69,77**	**12**	**27,91**
Progesterone 42 ewes	I	42	2	4,76	40**	95,24	2	9,52	17	40,48
	II	40	21	21,43	19	45,24	16	73,7	5	9,52
	III	24	22	4,76	2	2,38	1	50,00	1	0,5
	Mating	28	x	x	x	x	15	53,57	13	46,43
	Final	**42**	**2**	**4,76**	**x**	**x**	**32**	**76,19**	**8**	**19,05**
Progesterone + SGn (R) 47 ewes	I	47	0	0	47**	100	4	8,51	43	17,02
	II	43	22	17,02	21	44,68	15	71,43	6 ***	12,77
	III	28	27	12,77	1	0	0	0	1	17,02
	Mating	28	x	x	x	x	14	50, 00	14	50
	Final	**47**	**6**	**12,77**	**x**	**x**	**33**	**70,21**	**8**	**17,02**

*   2 ewes

**   3 ewes

*** 6 ewes were inseminated for the first time one ovarian cycle later.

In all three lots final low conception rates were registered. That could be explained by the fact that ewes without lamb in the spring were used in experiment. Very low conception rate were registered after artificial insemination in the first synchronized estrus cycles. That could be due to mistakes in semen processing in that days because much better conception rates were obtained also by artificial insemination in the next cycle of the same ewes. No doubt it was something wrong with the ewes' gynecology since the highest conception rate after free natural mating was 50%. The presented experiments argue for god results of estrus synchronization by using daily 10 mg of injecting progesterone treatment. Since infertility cases have a larger incidence in the control lot (27,91%) than in the experimental lots (19,05% in the experimental I and 17,02 in the experimental II lot) we think there is no negative action of progesterone treatment inducing anestrous state in ovary function. The 9 final real anestrous cases were present before treatment and that demonstrates the possible uterus infections in ewes.

But to have estrus synchronization each ewe has to be caught for at least 18 times (for 16 days of treatment and other 2 days for insemination). It is true that for insemination there is no reason to detect heat and perform blind insemination.

Nevertheless all ewes have to be caught and inseminate for 3 or 4 subsequent days.

Solution to avoid the waste of labor is given by progesterone impregnated intravaginali pessaries. One special experiment using Synchro-mate product was organized in the next year with the same kind of ewes on this target.[30] The experiment engaged 2 lots of ewes. The control lot didn't receive any treatment. The experimental lot received Synchro-mate pessaries for 19 days. That means 2 days more than 17 days indicated in the medicine prospect. This was decided because in the first four days after pessaries implementation ewes in heat have been discovered. In the 19th day from implementation, when pessaries were extracted, 800 IU of serum gonadotrophin (Roussel) was injected to every ewe. The graphs in the *figures 3.5* and *3.6* compare results of the two procedures of estrus synchronization in sheep at the beginning of the estrus season.

---

[30] Paraschivescu, M.; Ionășescu, L. *Utilization of "Synchromate" for the synchronization of heat in sheep mating season.* G.D.Searle London, 1967

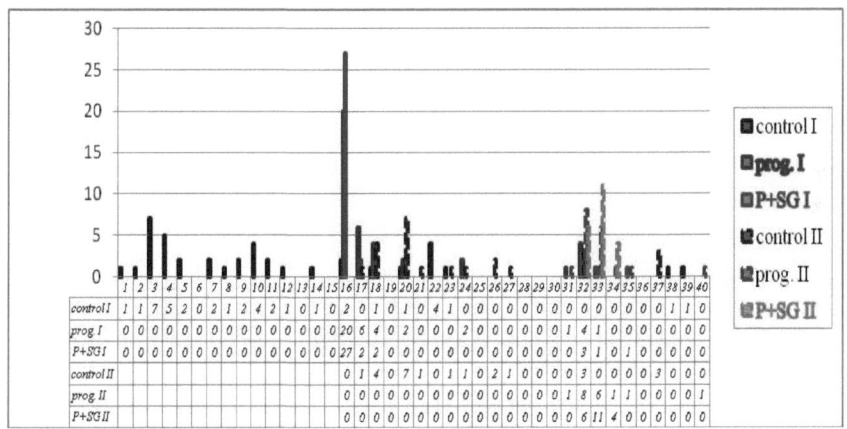

Fig.3.5. Estrus synchronization with progesterone injection

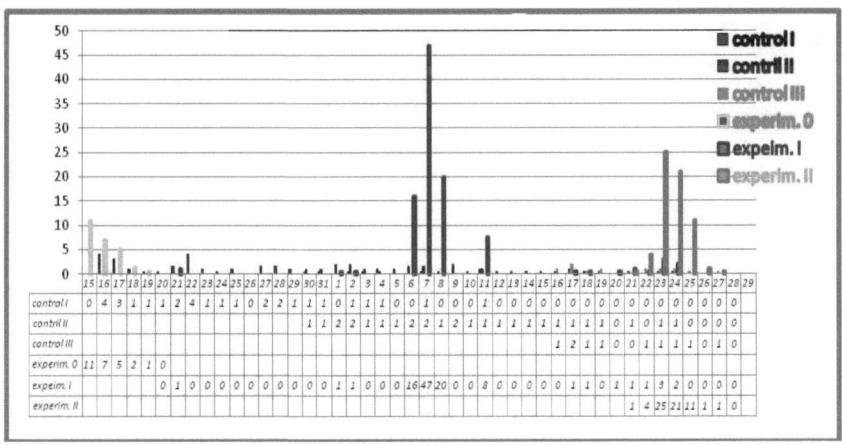

Fig.3.6. Estrus synchronization with Synchro-mate pessaries

In the last experiment the ewes in the control lot have shown the first heat starting with August 16. The last ewe with the first heat was registered in September 11. They return in heat starting with August 30, after 15 days from the first heat. The third cycle started 17 days later in August 16. In the experimental lot ewes in heat were found for 4 days the necessary time for progesterone absorption to start. Massive entrance in heat was registered after 21 days from the day of Synchro-mate pessaries implementation. In this interval of time 3 cases of heat were detected one of was a one day delayed progesterone absorption and the cases in September 1 and September 2, at 16 and 17 days form pessaries implementation where, may be, the vaginal walls didn't adhere to the pessaries to collect the necessary secretions for progesterone absorption. Other way as results from the presented graphs there is a high similitude between results of using estrus synchronization using Synchro-mate pessaries or daily progesterone injection. Both of them could be used for blind insemination at first heat after treatment. In addition using pessaries cases of metritis can be discovered. Then cumulated secretions in the ewe's vagina have unpleasant smell. Chronogest implant is also very good if implants can be extracted at term.

Diestrus interruption by yellow bodies' lysis has appeared when the Swedish research officer von Euler started to search for the presence in the prostate's secretion of boar of a factor helping fertilization of ova by sperms nobody has imagined a whole coordinating system of mammal animals' physiology will be discovered. Among the tissue hormones of this system, called prostaglandins but secreted by many tissues, Prostaglandin $F_{2\alpha}$ (PG $F_{2\alpha}$), secreted by the empty uterus, was found to be able to cause luteal body lysis. That was the beginning of a new modality of inducing estrus in puberty females at the wanted time. Of course action has started with the cow, the most important farm animal, and it was established that prostaglandin becomes active from the sixth day after estrus when the yellow body is wholly installed. It was also established that heat are expressed after 72 hours from PG $F_{2\alpha}$ administration. Parenteral intra muscular administration became satisfactory when Cloprostenolul was synthesized. Finally it was concluded that estrus synchronization of a whole group of puberty females requires two inoculations at 11 days interval have to be given.

But 11 days is the half of the 21 days cycle in cattle so we decided to use an 8 days interval in sheep, which is the half of the 17 days cycle in ewes. In order to find out what time $PGF_2\alpha$ becomes active in inducing heat and to know if there is any difference in prostaglandin action on the diestrus yellow body and pregnancy yellow body before embryo implementation, we organized one experiment on ewes of the local Tzurcana breed.[31] The experiment started in September 21 with estrus detection in a big flock. Each day ewes were marked to know the day of the estrus and one ewe was mated and the next one was not. Two experimental lots have been obtained one formatted from mated ewes and one formatted from non mated ewes. In the 12th day all the ewes received one doze of Flavoliz (a Na cloprostenol compound) recommended by its prospect.

---

[31] Paraschivescu, M.; Dinu, Cristina; Popa, I. *Efectul prostaglandinei asupra corpului galben de călduri și corpului galben de gestație la oile Țurcană.* Analele IBNA, vol.XVII, 1995

Ewes of both lots were controlled for heat with aproned teaser rams. Response to treatment is given in *Table 3.4*. Results were compared to the hypothetical reaction curve to prostaglandin and are presented in the *Fig.3.7*.

Table 3.4.

Answer of ewes' ovary to the PGF₂α in the first 11 days of the estrus cycle

days from estrus		1	2	3	4	5	6	7	8	9	10	11
hypothetical in heat		0	0	0	8	8	8	8	8	8	8	8
no mate	treated	10	15	12	10	18	13	10	10	10	8	7
	answered	0	0	0	1	5	2	1	4	4	7	3
	%	0	0	0	10		15	10	40	40	87,5	42,9
mated	treated	9	16	11	10	19	12	10	9	10	9	6
	answered	0	0	0	2	0	3	4	4	3	7	4
	%	0	0	0	20	0	25	40	44,4	30	77,8	66,7
total	treated	19	31	23	20	37	25	20	19	20	17	13
	answered	0	0	0	3	5	2	5	8	7	14	7
	%	0	0	0	15	13,5	8	20	42,1	35	82,4	53,8

The curve of coming in heat before treatment of ewes moves over and under the line of hypothetical mean of daily entrance of ewes in heat. That means the flock was in full sexual season when detecting heat was started, but the answer to the PGF₂α's treatment is under the hypothetical curve. Nevertheless certainly no ewe will react to the prostaglandin treatment in the first three days after estrus. Increasing tendency of reaction frequency of the yellow bodies to prostaglandin is registered. The peak of the curve's reaction in the 10th day after estrus is placed. No significant difference of yellow bodies' reaction in mated or non mated ewes has been registered.

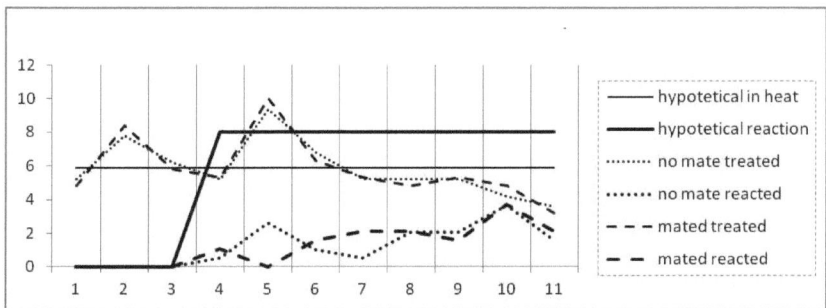

Fig.3.7. Reaction to the PGF₂α in the first 11 days of the estrus cycle

We disposed of this information when our research team tried to increase the fertility of one recently imported Corriedale sheep flock. Since the presence of the yellow body wasn't possible to be upholding by clinical means we have tried to discover cycling ovaries by coming in heat of ewes after prostaglandin treatment.[32] Such experiment was organized in a third Corriedale flock, disposing of three medicines based on cloprostenol (Flavoliz K based on cloprostenol K; Revoliz K based on D cloprostenol K and Revoliz Na based on D cloprostenol Na). Doses indicated by the products' instructions have been used at intervals of 8 days between inoculations. For heat detection aproned teaser rams have been used. Results are presented in *table 3.5.*

Table 3.5
Results of inducing heat by luteolysis

Kind of treatment	After first PGF			After second PGF			After 1+2		After third PGF			After 2+3	
	treated	reacted		treated	reacted		reacted		treated	reacted		reacted	
	No	No	%	No	No	%	No	%	No	No	%	No	%
Flavoliz K	50	27	54,0	23	17	73,9	44	88,0	6	1	16,7	18	78,3
Revoliz K	51	31	61,9	20	16	80,0	47	92,0	4	3	75,0	19	95,0
Revoliz Na	51	31	61,9	20	16	80,0	47	92,0	4	1	25,0	17	85.0
Total	152	89	58,6	63	49	77,8	138	90,8	14	5	35,7	54	85,7

All 152 of ewes were inoculated once. They were controlled for heat in the first 3 days after inoculation. The number of second treated ewes (in the table) represents the ewes that didn't show heat after the first treatment and received the second injection after 8 days. The third treatment was applied only to the ewes which haven't expressed heat after the 2 former treatments. They were considered as having a delayed sexual season. Finally 9 ewes (5,92%) didn't show heat because of prolonged anestrous. But if the term when yellow bodies react to prostaglandins is shorter than 8 days it is possible to have no response to prostaglandin in cycling ovaries as well.

In order to clarify the question we made this reasoning: We knew from former our search that the estrus cycle in Corriedale sheep has a medium length of 16 days and the estrus phase of the cycle is of 30 hours, as a mean. From this experiment resulted that for 138 eves reacting by heat after the two firsts treatments with prostaglandin that 89 ewes (64,49 %) have shown heat after the treatment applied in the 8th day of the cycle. Then in the first day of the cycle if no treatment is applied we must have 7,81% (100 %: 16 days x 1,25 for 30 hours

[32] Dinu, Cristina; Paraschivescu, M.; Szabo, I. *Controlul situaţiei ginecologice în sezonul de montă prin prostaglandine, la oile Corriedale.* Analele IBNA, vol.XVIII, 1995

length of the estrus) of ewes in heat, up to the 8th day of the cycle 64,49 % of ewes enter in heat and up to the 16th day of the cycle 100% of ewes are showing heat.

The equation of the regression line is of the type: $y = ax + b$

The values of a, which measures the flop of the regression line and of b result from fig.3.8.

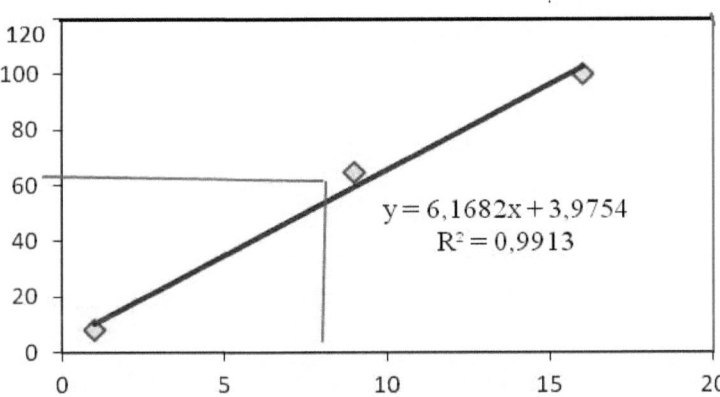

$$y = 6,1682x + 3,9754$$
$$R^2 = 0,9913$$

Fig.3.8. Regression line of yellow bodies' answer to prostaglandin

For the 9th day of the estrus the relation becomes:

$$64,49 = 6,1682x + 3,9754$$

$$x = \frac{64,49 - 3,9754}{6,1682} = 9,81$$

Since 9,81 days presence of active yellow body in the ovary is longer than the 8 days interval between prostaglandin injections that means any injected ewe might answer to prostaglandin treatment.

Synthetic lambing results are presented in Table 3.6. They allowed us to estimate mean number of estrus cycles per lambing.

Table 3.6.
Lambing results

Treatment	Treated heads	Ewes detected in heat	Ewes with lambs from:			Non parturient ewes		Remarks
			AI	B AI	NM	No.	%	
I	152	89	41	20	10	18	20,22	1,56 estrus cycles
II	63	48	12	11	3	22	45,83	1,65 estrus cycles
III	14	9	4	1	2	2	22,22	1,71 estrus cycles
Total	x	*146	57	32	15	42	28,76	1,60 estrus cycles

*Note: 4 ewes never showed heat; 2 ewes had delayed lambing from natural mating.

The global conception rate of the ewes responding to treatment was 104 lambing out of 146 ewes expressing heat what means 71,23 %.

The lowest conception rate, 0,26 %, was registered after final natural mating. The quota of non parturient 28,76% + 2,63% (4 permanently anestrous ewes) denotes acclimatization problems. These refer to hypothalamus function even photoperiodism is similar to the one of New Zeeland. Or maybe they are due to the stress caused by the grouped grazing system practiced in Romania.

Additional means to help estrous synchronization in ewes

The data in *table 3.6* suggest that in Corriedale sheep acclimatization process to the north latitude of Romania is not successful even photoperiodism control of the sexual activity in ewes must be similar to the one in New Zealand. The presence of without estrus ewes all over the autumn and the short length of the sexual season (we have registered the phenomenon in one other flock as well) suggests deficiencies in the ovary's function.

Then in order to find the cause of ovarian deficiencies a new experience with Corriedale sheep, using natural mating was organized.[33] If the functional deficiency of the ovary is due to an under normal follicular maturation and FSH is inoculated without any effect then it means that the ovarian structures are responsible for the noticed deficiencies. But if the deficiencies are corrected it means that the ovary doesn't receive enough FSH from the pituitary gland.

In this case there are two possibilities or the gland doesn't secret the gonadotrophin or the hormone is not released from the gland because hypothalamus doesn't emit enough GnRH. The experiment used 3 lots of ewes the E_1 what received Foligon (PMSGn) in the 14th day of the cycle, the lot C what received no treatment and the E_2 lot what received Fertagyl (GnRH) in the 15th day of the cycle. All of the ewes were naturally mated when were discovered in heat. Results are presented in *table 3.7*.

---

[33] Paraschivescu, M.; Gherciu, Mihaela; Dinu, Cristina; Nițulescu, Aneta; Murat, I. *Observații privind desfășurarea reproducției prin montă naturală.* Analele IBNA, vol.XVI,1993

Table 3.7.

Effects of PMSGn (Foligon) and GnRH (Fertagil) after mating, at the end of the ovary cycle

Lots	First cycle				Second cycle				Third cycle			Late lambing	Final	
	mounted	fertilized	returned	anestrous	mounted	fertilized	returned	anestrous	mounted	fertilized	anestrous		lambing	infertile
Foligon	45	22	22	1	22	15	2	6	2	2	6	0	39	6
Control	51	17	22	12	22	10	2	22	0	0	22	2	29	22
Fertagil	45	25	14	6	14	11	3	6	0	0	6	3	39	6

Final results show an increased effect of fertility when the ovary has been stimulated directly with the like FSH hormone from Foligon or indirectly with GnRH from Fertagyl, what realized FSH from the pituitary gland.

The same results are discussed, as percentage values, with the help of the graphic in *Fig.3.9.*

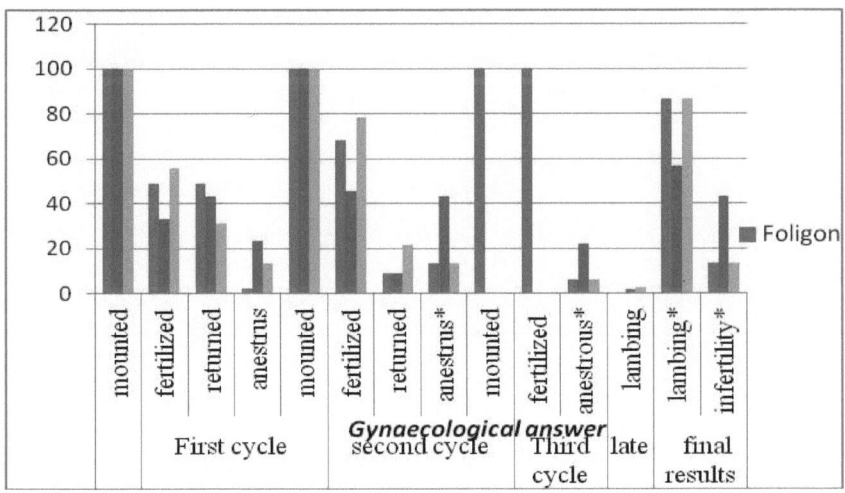

Fig.3.9. Ovary stimulation with PMSGn or GnRH

The percentage of ewes giving birth to lamb was equal in both lots of treated ewes (86,67%) much higher than in the control lot (64,44%). In the first ovarian cycle no ewe was treated. That means the lesser percent of coming in heat ewes was occasional. It was compensate by a higher number of cycling ewes in the time of second estrus cycle. In this cycle marked effect has the like FSH hormone. Thus 44 ewes out of 45 (97,78%) came in heat. It is a strong argument the ovary is a fully functional organ, able to answer to hormonal stimuli. Indirect stimulation of pituitary gland has less or no success in follicular stimulation but increased the rate of conception. High percent of ewes with lamb in the Fertagyl lot might be explained by a better conception rate due to more LH realized from the pituitary gland after GnRH injection. The absence of follicular stimulation could result of to a late administration of the realizing hormone. If so it is pituitary gland is completely functional and the ovary insufficiency is due to the hypothalamus, whose activity is related to optical stimuli. From the biotechnical point of view conclusion was both Foligon and Fertagyl help inducing heat al the desired term.

In the next autumn a new experiment to understand how GnRH is better to be used a new experiment was conceived.[34] Starting with September 24 ewes were controlled for heat. The ewes discovered in heat were mated and were distribute randomly in 4 lots. The first lot, the control one, received no treatment. The second one received 1doze of Fertagyl immediately when mated. The ewes in the third lot were mated and marked to recognize the day of showing heat and each of them received a dose of Fertagyl in the 15th day from the day when they have been mated. The ewes in the forth lot were mated and Chronogest pessaries were introduced in vagina to act as a yellow body for 15 days. The operation has been done since 38 ewes entered each lot. Results were analyzed in the spring estimating the conception rate of lots by the birth of lambs. These data are presented in *table 3.8*. The medium conception rate of the estrous cycles, as periods, were 66, 4 ± 3, 85 and, respectively 54, 3 ± 7, 02. These values and the conception rates per lots in the first two estrus cycles are presented in *Fig. 3.10*.

Table 3.8.

Fertagyl's action

Lots		Control		Fertagyl day 1		Fertagil day 15		Chronogest	
		number	%	number	%	number	%	number	%
cycle 1	heads	36	100	32	100	34	100	32	100
	births	21	58,3	24	75	24	70,6	21	65,6
cycle 2	heads	15	100	8	100	10	100	11	100
	births	5	33,3	5	62,5	6	60,0	6	54,5
cycle 3	heads	10	100	3	100	4	100	5	100
	births	3	30	0	0	0	0	0	0
total	births	29	80,6	29	90,6	30	88,2	29	85,3
	empty	7	19,4	3	9,4	4	11,8	5	14,7

---

[34] Dinu, Cristina; Paraschivescu, M.; Caproşu, V. *Durata sezonului de montă la oile Corriedale şi implicaţiile acesteia în reproducţie*. Zilele Cercetării Ştiinţifice, ICPCOC Palas, 1994

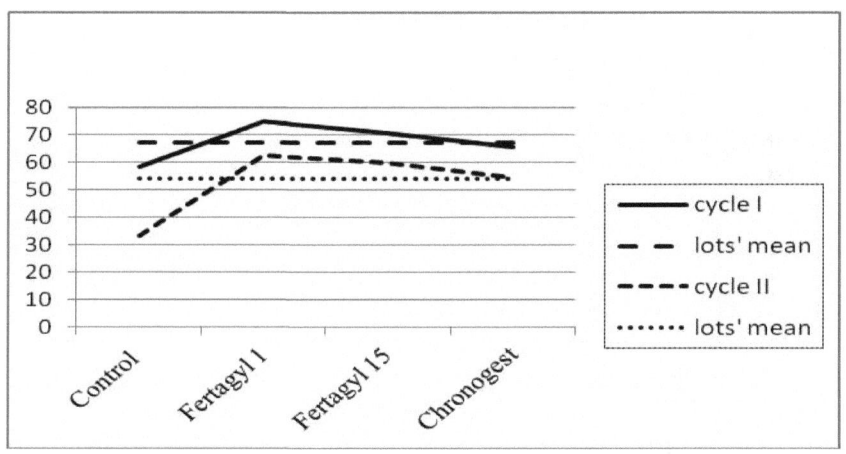

Fig.3.10. GnRH in the first and the fifteenth day of the estrous cycle

The lot receiving Fertagyl when mated registered highest conception rate in the spring. Difference is significant. That must be result of the LH released after GnRH from Fertagyl.

The lot receiving Chronogest registered better conception rate than the control lot but the difference is not significant. Using Fertagyl in the 15th day of the ovarian cycle didn't cause abortions and the conception rate was rather good. Perhaps the realized LH at this time reduced the number of ovular abortions since the elongation of the blastocist start after 12 days from the ovum's fertilization.[35]

In the period of the second ovarian cycle conception rate of the control lot decreased significantly related to acclimatization, may be. The highest conception rate (62,5) is again in the lot of ewes which have received Fertagyl in the first day after mating. Explanation of the fact could be that the realized FSH after GnRH in Fertagyl has stimulated the maturation of the new follicular wave in the ovaries of the non fertilized ewes. Similar conception rate (60,0%) has been registered in the lot of ewes receiving Fertagyl in the 15th day of the cycle. Intravaginali inserted Chronogest pessaries helped the conception rate after their removal but less than the Fertagyl inoculation. Double Fertagyl administration

---

[35] Paraipan, V. *Hormonoterapia la animalele domestice.* Editura Agrosilvică, 1982

in the first and the fifteenth day after ewes' inseminations could be usefully in blind artificial insemination of ewes after estrus synchronization of heat with prostaglandins.

Estrous synchronization outside of the mating season

Usually out of the mating season ewes are in anestrous state. That means neither antral follicles nor active luteal bodies are present in ovaries of not pregnant ewes. We will call these ewes "empty". We can't call them "dry" because dry refers to the udder. We can't call them "barren" because they are able to conceive and become pregnant after treatment.

There are flocks or even breeds able to be mated and be fertilized in the spring and have lamb in autumn. In spring biotechnologically interest is to increase heat incidence or/and to synchronize estrous for blind artificial insemination. For these two goals used the opportunity of disposing in Palas Research Station of Romania of a flock of empty ewes, non pregnant and without lambs in the spring. Part of them had the former lambing in autumn and part of them had it in spring. We have separated them in two flocks. In the first flock ewes were included if their previous lambing was in spring. In the second flock ewes with the previous lambing in autumn were included. In each of the flocks 3 three experimental lots were randomly formatted: the first lot received parenteral 10 mg of progesterone daily during 16 days. The second one received the same progesterone treatment and in addition 350 IU of PMSGn. Associated to the last dose of progesterone. The third acted as control lot and received no treatment.[36]

The graph *(Fig.3.11.)* shows higher heat incidence and better estrous synchronization after treatment in the flock having the former lambing in spring. Association of PMSGn to Progesterone increased a little bit the heat incidence in the flock and shortened the proestrus phase of the estrous cycle.

---

[36] Paraschivescu, M.; Ursescu, Al. *Ovarian stimulation in sheep out of the estrus season.* G.D.Searle London 68, 1967

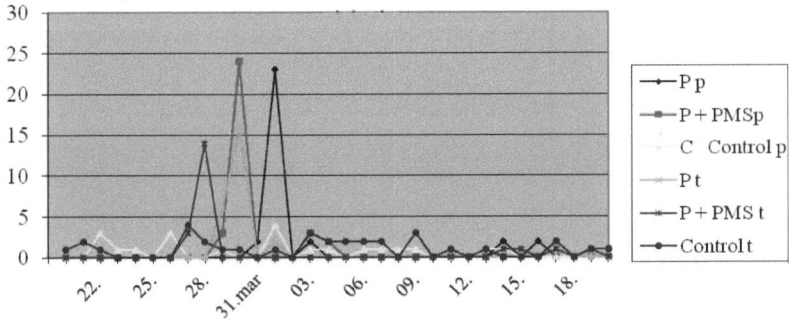

Fig.3.11. Estrus synchronization in the spring using progesterone parental injection

In the flock with the former lambing in autumn PMSGn has shortened the proestrus phase as well but didn't increased estrus synchronization.

From the *table 3.9* it results that heat incidence was higher (83,6%) in the control lot with the former lambing in autumn than in the control lot (77,8%) with ewes having the former lambing in spring. At the same time the response of ewes to the hormonal treatment was much better in ewes with a cycling ovary in the previous spring. So 100% of the ewes with former lambing in autumn treated with PMSGn associated to progesterone entered in heat, compared to 65,2% of ewes with the former lambing in spring.

Table 3.9.
Estrus synchronization out of sexual season in relation with the season of the former lambing

Former lambing	Treatment	Total		In heat		Returned		Fertilized		Final fertility		Twins	
		No	%	No	%	No	%	No	%	No	%	No	%
spring	P	44	100	31	70,8	3	9,7	10	32,3	10	32,3	2	20
	P+PMS	49	100	32	65,2	4	12,5	8	25,0	22	68,8	11	50
	Control	35	100	27	77,8	6	22,2	9	33,3	16	59,3	9	56,2
autumn	P	25	100	23	93,4	2	8,7	7	30,4	14	60,9	0	0,0
	P+PMS	20	100	20	100,0	4	20,0	12	60,0	12	60,0	5	41,7
	Control	37	100	31	83,6	2	5,4	12	38,7	15	48,4	3	20,0

Relevant difference exists between the lot treated with progesterone alone (93,4% versus 70,8%). From the same table it is seen that the number of returned ewes in heat after the first mating and the number of fertilized ewes after the first mating is much lower than the mated ewes in the first ovarian cycle, doesn't matter if the estrus was natural or induced by the treatment. Exception is shown only by the lot of ewes with the previous lambing in autumn that received PMSGn after progesterone where there a good conception rate was registered. That demonstrates a short length of the individual sexual activity in the spring. The same conclusion is given by the final fertility registered in both of the control lots. Acceptable final fertility resulted in the two lot receiving PMSGn, together with a higher incidence of birth with twins.

The servitude of the presented above experiment is the great amount of labor needed for the progesterone treatment. We mounted a new experiment[37] in the same location using a lot that received intravaginali Cronolone impregnated pessaries for 16 days associated with 350 IU of PMSGn inoculated in the day when pessaries have been extracted. The heat incidence was 83,3% in the experimental lot and 84,1% the control one. The treatment didn't increase heat incidence in the treated flock but determined satisfactory estrus synchronization. After 24 hours since pessaries have been extracted 69,2% of ewes entered in heat within 2 days. The graph of heat expression presented in *Fig.3.12* demonstrates it. The PMSGn treatment increased the conception rate by 8,8% and the frequency of births with twins by 8,0%.

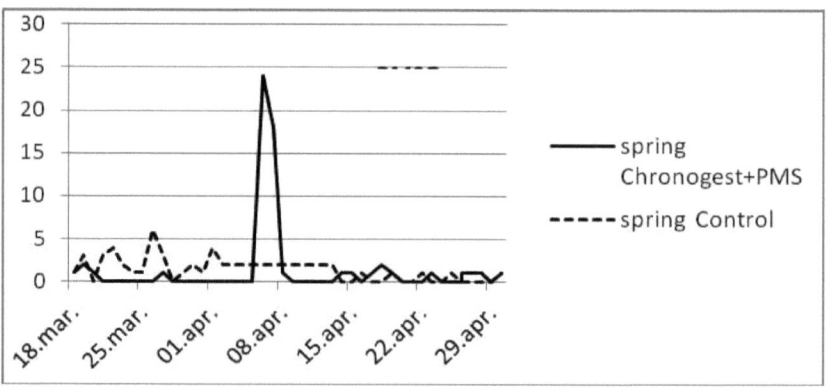

Fig.3.12. Estrous synchronization in spring with Chronoone - PMSGn

[37] Paraschivescu, M.; Ursescu, Al. *Influenţarea vieţii sexuale la ovine în sezonul de primăvară prin tratamente hormonale.* Lucrările Congresului Internaţional de Biologie a Reproducţiei, Moscova, 1966

Following the above experiments we can admit the tendency of repeating the ovarian ciclicity out of season once it was induced. That explain why it was possible to create breeds like the German breed Merinolandschaf able to have the sexual season in the spring.

In other breeds out of season estrus synchronization requires a substitute hormonal treatment starting with vaginal insertion of Chronolone pessaries or under skin Chronogest implants for at least 9 days and associate 350 IU of PMSGn one day before pessaries or implants extraction or 600 IU of FSH in the day of extraction, as under skin injection. Better synchronization is obtained if in the previous day of the above treatment an active doze of prostaglandin is injected intramuscularly.

Super ovulation is controlled as well using FSH of ovine or porcine origin in three days before proestrus or with one dozes of 350 IU of PMSGn immediately before proestrus. Proestrus is obtained when controlled diestrus is deblokate, in sexual season, or at the end of a complete substitute hormonal treatment when the action is provided out of the mating season.

Multiple ovulation in sense of collecting embryos by repeating super ovulation is provided only once at the next estrus cycle after embryo washing. That could be explained by the little number of ovarian cycles during the sexual season or may be because before embryos have been collected surgically.

In vitro fertilization (IVF) and advanced genomic biotechnologies

In vitro fertilization is the biotechnology permitting access the ova or the zygote before ova fertilization. That allows foreign DNA sequences of very different genetic species, even vegetal ones, to be transferred in sheep embryos. Transfer of DNA sequence can be done mechanically by injecting the foreign DNA into the male pronuclee that is larger, but is preferred both pronuclee to be injected. Biding the DNA sequence to a virus vector and injecting it in the ovum cytoplasm gives chance both pronuclee to be penetrated and to have a more efficient gene transfer. Electro porous techniques exercised in plant aren't necessary.

The male genomic structures are placed in sperms. Artificial insemination in sheep seldom uses fresh semen. Long term preservation of semen is ensured by freezing. Time ago semen was processed in pellets form by CO_2 dry ice. Now straws and liquid Nitrogen are preferred.

The most interesting biotechnology with sperms is to determine the spermatozoon's sex using fluorescent in situ hybridization (FISH)[38] in order to control the sex of the progeny. Embryo sexing in breeding flocks seems to be illogical. More female progeny will speed increasing the population breeding stock but will decrease selection intensity of male genitors whose contribution to genetic progress of population is much greater than the females' one. More male progeny will increase selection intensity of sires but will send to slaughter house a larger number of animals before producing anything else then body gain. On the other hand in present time the method is laborious and costly.

The female genomic structures are placed in ovules. Ovules are used for in vitro fertilization (IVF). These techniques allow access to the zygote structures. On this basis transgenic organisms carrying foreign DNA have been obtained.[39] This is a very important fact for pharmaceutics industry. The DNA sequence transferred commands syntheses of a protein of interest. Usually the trangenesis success is recognized by the presence of transferred genes in the milk of genetically modified organism obtained. In this respect ewes are preferred since they are less costly than cows or goats. In this case only fertilized eggs by X chromosome sperm are of interest for the enzyme's production. Sexing transgenic embryos is wanted since female transgenic organisms secreting milk are preferred. Nevertheless transgenic "male" embryos are of interest for a further sexual reproduction of transgenic pairs. Meanwhile success of transgenesis is not always certain and its diagnosis is difficult especially in males. Therefore is hard to format pairs of transgenic animals in order to sexually reproduce them less costly. More than that during gametes' meiosis there is chance adduced genes to be eliminated when the embryo's genome is formatted.

Diploid genomes are in fertilized ova. Reproduction biotechnologies work with embryos before hutching out of *zona pellucida*.

Long term conservation of embryo by freezing is a solved question.[40] The lent (English method) freezing, the rapid freezing or the vitrification freezing are applied with satisfactory results. The most used crioprotectoare is glycerin. We

---

[38] Mateescu, Raluca *Marker Assisted Selection in Animal Breeding*. Training course at Animal Biology and Nutrition Institute, Bucharest, Romania, 2011
[39] Zamfirescu, Stela; Şonea, Al. *Biotehnologii de Reproducere la Rumegătoarele Mici*. ISBN: 973-644-113-X, Editura ExPonto, 2004
[40] Willadsen, S.M.; Polge, C.; Rowson, L.E.A.; Moor, R.M. *Deep freezing of sheep embryos*. Journal of Reproduction and Fertility 46, 1976

have no experience in using the etillen glycol crioprotector in sheep. The success rate of embryo transfer goes up to 60%.

Ruther successful attempts have been made to have twins from receptors females out of embryo transfer. Better results are wanted concerning the fertilization rate of super ovulated ova in order to increase the number of transferable embryos before freezing them. Better synchronization of the gynecological state of receptor ewes with the age of the transferred embryos is also desired.

Embryo splitting could be solution to increase fertility of donor ewes. We have receipt very interesting information (from a Canadian veterinarian) that the coat of twins resulting from embryo splitting differs, even the biochemical indices are similar. That means that the skin traits are very early established.

Diploid genomes (somatic cells' nuclei) are used to obtain *clones* of mammal animals. Cloning of sheep organism has been successfully provided. Important condition is to have a good synchronization of the transferred nucleus division phase with the division phase of the ovum nucleus. In this respect we have to remember the famous Dolly case. Now it is said some hundreds of clones of Dolly's type have been obtained. In this case clones have been obtained from adult somatic cells, but clones can be obtained from embryonic cells, too. Cloning of mammals is very important for transgenic animals' reproduction. Superior animals' cloning from adult cells is a very important fact for pharmaceutical industry since it gives the possibility to reproduce transgenic organisms without sexual reproduction.

Chimeras occur when foreign blastomeres were implanted in the germinal disc of one embryo of the same genetic species. The foreign traits expressed by chimeras are not reproduced in their progeny. We didn't any experiment with chimeras.

*

Concerning IVF and embryo transfer in sheep hopes for the future are connected to improving the endoscope technique of collecting embryos in order to save the life of genetically valuable donors. There are also hopes to increase the fertilization rate of super ovulated ova by improving the inseminated spermatozoa capacitating.

Chapter 4
DISCLOSING OUTPUTS OF SHEEP BREEDING BY BIOTECHNOLOGIES

Concept

Estimating the undemonstrative spare outputs of sheep breeding disclosed by reproduction and genomic biotechnologies in sheep breeding pretends much imagination because of the multitude of known procedures and because of the diversity of products obtained from sheep flocks.

Generally speaking sheep farming aims to offer for the market goods in order to get profit. The profit level depends on the relation existing for each product between the price per unit of product and the cost of the same unit. A good price of product is obtained when the product is much required and small quantities of it are offered by producers.

The output of sheep farms is given by the obtained price per product unit and by the quantity of produced goods doesn't matter if they were sold or not yet. Costs are classified in variable costs which modifies together with the produced quantity of goods, fixed costs, which are inherent for production and maintain their level even the production is stopped, and added fixed costs as taxes, publicity or other expenses of the kind which have no contribution to the quantity nor to the quality of the goods produced.[41]

The difference between the total output and the variable costs is giving the farm gross margin. It must be positive to start a business. The farm gross margin minus the fixed costs gives the farm profit or loss. That is the gross profit. The gross profit minus the added fixed costs gives the net profit of the farm. Farmers can influence the quantity of produced goods and the variable costs per unit of product.

In order to measure value each country uses its currency. There is an each day currency quotation changing the quotas of peculiar currencies. Prices are frequently changing with the offer and require of the market. That modifies the level of costs as well. For these reasons the authors of this study will try to avoid using the Romanian currency in the economic analysis of reproduction biotechnology effect in sheep breeding. They will to imagine peculiar analyses

---

[41] Paraschivescu, M.Th. *Studiu de proiect privind înființarea unei ferme MOET cu circuit deschis.* Teză de Doctorat, U.S.A.M.V.București, 2002

for each case of practicing reproduction biotechnologies in known farming conditions.

Considering the complexity of the present theme our study will discuss the diversity of goods produced with the sheep related specie's biodiversity, will underline the effect of peculiar reproduction biotechnologies upon the quantity of ware disposed for the market and will suggest opportunities to use them in order to disclose undemonstrative outputs of sheep flocks, based on their former experiments.

Among the domesticated animal genetic species, sheep is the one giving the most diversified kind of goods. Sheep are producing wool, at list three kinds of wool related to the fiber diameter: thin wool ($< 24\mu$), meddle wool ($28\mu - 36\mu$) and thick wool ($> 37\mu$). There is also white wool and colored wool. Related to the wool production there are breeds covered with the denomination of Merino Sheep. The most famous breed is the Australian Merino. A preserved old breed is the Rambouilet Merino, in France. There are also Merino breeds in Spain (as native breeds), in some European countries including Romania, in Russia and in other countries having dry climate. Implication of reproduction biotechnologies in thin wool production could be blind artificial insemination using purebred rams of thin fiber. Unfortunately wool is not enough appreciated, now days, except in Australia. That means there is no desire to increase wool production in other countries except the Russian Federation.

Sheep are producing meat. There are at least three kinds of sheep meat. The Mouton, what is a lean meat obtained mostly from young animals grown up to 30 -35 kg of body weight. This kind is required in Western European counties and other countries undertaken English influence. Countries having dry climate and low vegetables' production, like Arabian countries or Mongolia prefer a fat mutton containing vitamins in their suet. There countries, like Romania, for instance, that prefer to consume sucking lambs. Producers' interests differ with kind of meat they intend to offer for market. In case of mutton production there is interest for more meaty carcasses from and for faster growing lambs from some local ewes. This goal can be hit with blind artificial insemination using fresh semen collection or preserved deep frozen semen. For good mutton English breed like Southdown, Suffolk, Romney Marsh, Lincoln, Leicester, Border Leicester and so on are appreciated. For fat carcasses the Romanian local breeds Tzurcana and Tzigaia are very good. The traditional pastoral farming system with the natural mating reproduction is the most convenient one. In the extensive pastoral farming system the goal of getting more sucking lambs to be slaughtered is not fulfilled by increasing the frequency of birth with twins because too much new borne lambs are lost. Biotechnologies of this kind may be applied in intensive farming system only. Twins aren't wanted in Karakul breed too, because lambs' pelts are of smaller size.

Milk production is desired especially in the undeveloped countries where the extensive farming is in use. Then good mobility of ewes is appreciated and has to be preserved. There is much need of labor in production of milk. Nevertheless new intensive farming for sheep milk production is going up now. Two specialized sheep breeds for milk production are in vogue. The Friesian breed, in Netherland, created for a humid climate and Awassy breed, in Israel, created for intensive farming in dry climate. A new breed is now days developing (in Palas Research Institute of Romania) able for as a long lactation period as to suppress the seasonal anestrous and continue in the mating season. In this breed ewes are pregnant and in milk at the same time.

Pelts from very young lambs are much appreciated. There are two kinds of wanted pelts. Karakul pelts on ringed fibers and "mouton d'auré "pelts prepared from young lambs skin of different middle fiber wool sheep. For this purpose large new born lambs are desired.

Skins of adult sheep are also wanted for covers or fur coats. A special quality is offered by the skin of Romanov sheep breed whose coat has shorter thick fibers and little longer thin ones. Such kind of skin is much appreciated in fur cups' manufacture. This kind of fur isn't possible to have from other breeds or crosses. The target of disclosing undemonstrative spare outputs by reproduction biotechnologies in sheep is very complex because of the great number of possible biotechnologies that could be used and the high diversity of possible goals to be attained in different farming systems.[42]

To pass over difficulties we will make an attempt to classify the main fields reproduction biotechnologies might be applied and to appreciate their specificity. The main fields are:

a) to get *genetic progress* of the breeding stock of pedigree animals selected to conceive in closed reproduction the new generations of pedigree animals of one sheep breed;

b) to improve the quality or to increase the quantity of products from a sheep flock with commercial purpose using crossbreeding;

---

[42] Paraschivescu, M.Th.; Paraschivescu, M.; Bogdan, A.T.; Tobă, G.F.; Sandu, Mariana; Ipate, Judith; Stan, Simona; Dobre, Dana. *Some aspects of farm animal biodiversity formation on Romania's actual teritory*. DAGENE, Hunedoara, 2010

c) to multiply transgenic organisms by cloning them from adult somatic cells;

d) to preserve *"ex situ"* breeds in critical state of extinction.

Getting genetic progress of breeding stock

Genetic progress refers to a selection criterion which can be one qualitative trait, a quantitative indicator or one selection index.[43] Continuous quantitative values must be used. In case of qualitative traits score scale are imagined in order to obtain continuous values. Selection efficiency decreases with the number of criteria included in one index as in the mathematical equation:

$$efficiency = \frac{1}{\sqrt{n}} \ (where \ n = the \ number \ of \ criteria)$$

In genetic evaluation of breeding animals is good distinguish between *genetic merit* and *genetic value*. Literature is not very clear in this respect. We prefer to consider *genetic merit* the measure (value) of selection criterion found in individuals. In many cases we have to appreciate the difference between the genetic merit given by the genotype and the genetic merit given by phenotype using the heritability coefficient. Meanwhile we consider *genetic value* the position of genetic merit in the population to which animal pertains concerning its place in the population hierarchy and inside its family. Many times *genetic value* is expressed as predicted difference and is quantified in percent units.

In grading up improvement of breeds better *genetic progress* can be obtained with higher selection intensity or with higher precision of selection. Higher selection intensity is possible when individual fertility of parents is increased. Precision of selection is the best when progeny's performances are considered but this procedure requires long generation interval. To this procedure someone can add ancestors' and sibs' performances to be improved. When selection decision is possible before puberty self performance test is preferred. This test can be improved adding ancestors' and sibs' performances, too. Now breeding organization are spiking about "animal model".

Artificial insemination is able to highly increase of rams' fertility. Thus AI permits to select with higher precision the best son of a ram when the selection criterion is appreciated on the sons when they have attained the puberty age. This is the case of mutton breeds, of thin or middle wool breeds or even of pelt Karakul breed. For the case of milk production where traits cannot be

---

[43] Voicu, Rita; Caproşu, A.; Paraschivescu, M.; Ghiţă, Elena. *Efectul selecţiei direcţionale consecutiv procedeelor de ameliorare în rasă curată a oilor Corriedale.* Anale IBNA, volum XVI,1993

appreciated on rams, a minimum number of 30 pairs daughter – contemporary are required and the AI becomes necessary. But using or not using the artificial insemination is a question of costs. Since AI is not expensive, it might be used to know the genetic abilities of rams in all of excellence flocks. Very interesting discoveries could be done by progeny test concerning the genotype of rams in Karakul flocks producing pelts of different colors. Thus pelts of wanted colors could be obtained at will, not by hazard. Blind artificial insemination has the merit of certainly known origin of animals. Using ET or other associated to ET technologies with the purpose to increase selection intensity for genetic progress seems to be too expensive. The question of progeny test of Karakul rams for color pelt genotype remains open since up to now no experiment on this purpose was imagined and provided.

Increasing the commercial value of farm outputs

Any shepherd wants to produce more for the market and to have better price for its products. At the same time he intends to have the least production costs and the best use of his farm resources. Let's say we are in a sheep farm in the mountain area of Romania, where pasture is poor and cool rains are frequent during summer time. He breeds sheep of the local Tzurcana breed of light animals, covered of thick wool coat, having fat carcasses and producing acceptable milk yield after lambs are weaned. Up to now things were good. Being light sheep could walk long distances to feed them self on poor pasture, having a thick wool coat they resisted to cool rains, consumers around liked to have a Easter lamb and preferred the sheep cheese versus the cow cheese. The fat carcass hasn't too much importance. It is used to prepare a special salt meat of local tradition or aged ewes are sold to retailers to be exported in Arabian countries.

Now mouton is required for good prices in Western Europe. He has to use British heavy mouton sheep breeds. But he is not stupid. He understands heavy mouton ewes aren't able to feed themselves walking on the poor mountain pasture he disposes of.

Then he could apply one crossbreeding program using rams of one British mouton breed. In this case half of his breeding ewes will be mated to mouton rams and will stay down in the home yard since lambs are weaned and move to the feed lot. All this progeny will be sold. The other half of ewes will be breed as it was usually bred. Lambs will be sold for the Easter and only the needed she lambs to replace the old ewes will be kept. Of course some male lambs will be retained for reproduction. But mouton rams are expensive. If they were used for one season only the full difference of price between the sum paid for a breeding ram and the money received when it is sold to the slaughter house must be distribute to let say 40 – 50 lambs.

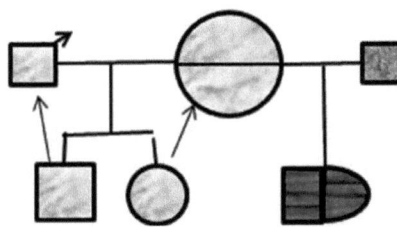

Fig.4.1. Model of crossbreeding program based on natural mating

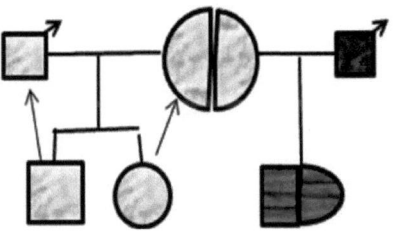

Fig.4.2. Model of crossbreeding program based on artificial insemination

If they are kept for the next mating seasons al costs of their feeding and housing have to be considered and they couldn't resist more than 3 seasons as a mean. Much cheaper is to claim for the biotechnology help and practice blind artificial insemination buying 2 doses of deep frozen semen of mouton rams and synchronizing heat with Chronogest under skin implants or Chronolone intravaginali pessaries and stimulating follicular stimulation with 300 -500 IU of PMSGn. In the second day after insemination the local rams will be introduced in the ewe flock for free mating or for former reproduction system. In the spring about 50% of the ewes will have cross lambs. These will be the first lambing ewes they will be isolated from the rest of the flock and will suckle the lambs for fast growing. May be many twin lambs will be registered as well. The other ewes will be moved to the mountain pasture and will be milked as before and will furnish the new generations of the breeding stock.

Let say other shepherd is located in the plain area, disposes of a better pasture and has a flock of Tzigaia sheep. This shepherd has to reject British mouton breeds because atmosphere humidity is to low and animals don't resist. This one can apply the same crossbreeding plan with artificial insemination. He can add the administration of one doses of PMSGn after 16 days from the previous doses in order to have more twins of Tzigaia breed. This time twins are desired because their mothers have to move less on pasture to feed themselves. If the mouton price is very good and his pasture is very reach this shepherd could use, after estrous synchronization without follicular stimulation, embryo transfer instead of artificial insemination. Transferring 2 embryos to each donor he might have higher benefit.

Let us now imagine another case. The shepherd is interested in producing more milk per ewe. A non genetic way la hit this target is to have longer lactation. Practicing the nearby scheme he can transfer to all ewes one Karakul embryo, instead of mouton sheep embryos. Half of his ewes will give birth to a lamb that will be scarified at 3 days of age and its mother yielded lactation will be at least one month longer. In addition these ewes will have a longer milking period based on the beginning of lactation when the daily milk yield is more. In this case the shepherded win the value of the pelts and the value of the plus o milk from the first about 45 days of lactation. It is for sure that the sum of the goods mentioned before goes over the costs of the embryo transfer.

If these scheme is applied in Karabasha flocks, the breed being known as giving birth to large lambs the value of pellets will be higher since from larger mothers are born larger progenies and the price of pelts are related to their surface. Or maybe if two embryos are transferred 2 good pelts would be obtained.

If the life of donors is saved when the embryo are washed, that will reduce the

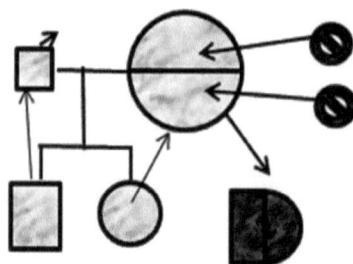

embryo transfer costs then more opportunities are opened in applying reproduction biotechnologies in sheep. In this case production of embryos has to be concentrated out of mating season of ewes. The main sources of added outputs are a higher fertility of ewes from induced by super ovulation twinning, eventually associated with higher commercial value of new born lambs, or by producing and saving embryos during the long anestrous

Fig.4.3 Model of breeding program based on multiple embryo transfer

between two pregnancies. Ewes' fertility could be increased by reducing the lambing interval. Two lambing per year is not excluded.

Controversies about artificial fertility in sheep are related to the farming system, to the intended product to be obtained and to the method of inducing higher artificial fertility.

Before discussing this question as a study case it is necessary to make clear some terms concerning reproduction in sheep. In the pre pubertal period of life the cyclic activity of the ovary is absent. It is generally accepted that there is a hormonal activity apart the ovary that induces the sexual dimorphism. Or perhaps the dimorphism is due to the presence in each cell of the body of the X chromosome whose action is not stopped by TDF, the factor contained by the Y chromosome that had differentiate the testis formation with their interstitial cells secreting the specific hormone of males. The ovarian "*acyclic state*" induces the lack of hormonal secretion of the ovary. Nor *estrogens* and nor *progesterone* are secreted. That is the *anestrous* state. It differs of *diestrus,* absence of sexual desire in mammal females due to the secretion of progesterone by the inner theca of ovarian follicles and of the yellow bodies formatted after ovulation. But *anestrous* exists from parturition up to the mating season, as it is shown in the *Fig.2.4.* Thus the usual fertility in sheep is one lamb per year and some cases of twin lambing.

Shepherds, in some circumstances by selection, managed to develop this trait and have created some prolific breeds as for instance Romanov breed in Russia, Finish Landrace in Finland, Borulla Merino in Australia and the Palas Prolific Breed in Romania. The fertility of these breeds is higher than the usual one and we will call it *natural fertility.*

Higher fertility might also be obtained by follicular stimulation to produce pollyovulation. We will call it *artificial fertility*. But there is another kind of artificial fertility that could be obtained by inducing heat and ovulation outside of the mating season decreasing inter lambing interval. This time the treatment must create, artificially, the full chain of hormonal control of the estrus cycle adding also the follicular stimulation for super ovulation.

We mentioned above that shepherds have created *natural fertility breeds* in some circumstances only, where they were interested to have it. In other circumstances they don't like higher fertility than the usual one. Artificial fertility is not always desired.

The pastoral extensive farming where flocks have to go long distances to feed themselves doesn't like twin lambing especially when ewes are milked.

Shepherds prefer stronger, mobile lambs that grow faster and can be weaned earlier. When ewes aren't milked, for instance in merino sheep, twins are desired (e.g. Borula Merino breed). I this last case if feeding resources don't differ during the year two parturitions per year might be desired.

In Karakul sheep twins are not wanted because they are smaller and depress the pellet price. Increasing fertility in sheep producing pellets by obtaining 2 parturitions per year is not convenient, too, because the value of milk could be higher than the value of the pellet. Generally speaking in milking ewes longer wet periods are preferred to shorter inter lambing intervals. It may be look strange but short inter lambing interval are wanted in prolific sheep bred in extensive farming.

Artificial fertility is desired in the intensive farming excepting the case of the milk production. High natural fertility is obtained by breeding, but this requires long time up to success. Artificial high fertility offer immediate results but has the servitude of costs. Costs include medicines, qualified labor and manipulation of animals. All projects of this kind have to be preceded by feasibility study.

Virtues and servitudes of MOET will be treated from the point of view of the needed reproduction services and from the point of view of commercial animal owners. Of course MOET virtues are expressed in case of breeds' transfer in new locations and perhaps to increase selection intensity in genetically active farm for mouton or milk. One avant-garde idea would be to imagine progeny test of rams for milk production, a challenge for MOET.

There are many chances of MOET success in sheep. The reason of this assertion is the high biodiversity of this genetic species, the seasonal sexual activity and the short pregnancy. The lambing interval is 365 days including a 148 days of pregnancy as a mean. The events of reproduction and the succession of gynecological states have been presented in *Fig 2.4.*

Ex situ biodiversity preservation

As it was explained before biodiversity conservation means to maintain the number of biological populations. This assertion is valuable both for nature and for culture. Concerning *"in situ"* farm animal conservation we must know it requires keeping in closed reproduction a sufficient number of animals, grouped in so many families as to be able to avoiding genetic drift. That is rather difficult from technical point of view, presents the risk of unwanted crossbreeding and is very costly. No private breeder will assume such costs just to hope for a perhaps future need for some preserved genes.

While in nature animals populations is accepted to be in critical states of extinction when they have less than 100 individual's contingency, in farm animals this state of risk depends on the generative precocity index in females, on the degree of accepted inbreeding and on the length of used puberty for breeding. The generative precocity index in sheep is 2 years, both for females or males, the accepted common ancestor may be placed in the third generation and the shortest term to use a ram is two years long in order to be sure having one male descendent of him. There is a need of at least 4 families in the flock each family being formatted of two rams and 12 ewes, 6 for the old ram from 3 different families. The distribution of ewes per families must be 1 ewe, the oldest one, from one family, 2 middle age ewes from other second family and 3 ewes, the youngest, pertaining to a third family. Ewes' families mustn't be common with the ram's family. The distribution of ewes for the young ram has to respect the same rule but the family of the same age must differ. All together the flock must be composed out of 8 rams and 96 ewes pertaining to 4 families.

The *"ex situ"* preservation of populations in critical states of extinction is a more convenient alternative to *"in situ"* preservation. Reproduction biotechnology with sheep could be based of deep freezing of semen or embryos. In case of a deep frozen depot of semen, haploid genomic information is used. Therefore rebuilding a breed *"in situ"* will require to use successive cross breeding using females of a local convenient breed for at least 7 generation (14 years) to have less than 1% foreign blood. Therefore rebuilding a breed *"in situ"* will require to use successive cross breeding for at least 7 generation to have less than 1% foreign blood, starting with females of a local convenient breed. In order to obtain a final convenient population de initial depot of semen must have semen from at least 4 rams which aren't relatives and to preserve about 12500 dozes of semen from each ram in order to have after 7 generations one initial population of 4 families with 2 rams and around 25 females per family.

But all these things are simple counting. The project of building up a sheep population out of a semen depot is not a very simple question. It is necessary to start the project 600 ewes of a loc al breed that we call it the "maternal breed". Accepting a conception rate of 50% out of artificial insemination in the first year we will dispose of 600 ewes to be inseminated giving birth to 150 young females able for reproduction after 2 years. In the second year we will have again the former 600 ewes to be inseminated. In the third year of the project the

600 of the maternal breed will be used again and in addition 150 F1 females will be inseminated. In the fourth year of the project the female breeding lot will consist out of the same 600 ewes of the maternal breed and now 300 F_1 generation females. In the fifth year of the project the female breeding lot will include 600 female of the maternal breed 450 females F1 and, for the first time, 38 F2 females. In order to press the implementation of the preserved breed starting with the sixth year using of the maternal breed has to be excluded. This year the female breeding stock will consist of 600 F1 females and 113 F2 females. Further insemination plan can be followed in *Table 4.1.*

Table 4.1.

Project to building up a sheep population from preserved deep frozen semen

Year	MB	F1	F2	F3	F4	F5	F6	F7	F8	Ewes
I	600	x	x	x	x	x	x	x	x	600
II	600	x	x	x	x	x	x	x	x	600
III	600	150	x	x	x	x	x	x	x	750
IV	600	300	x	x	x	x	x	x	x	900
V	600	450	38	x	x	x	x	x	x	1088
VI	0	600	113	x	x	x	x	x	x	713
VII	0	750	225	10	x	x	x	x	x	985
VIII	0	600	375	38	x	x	x	x	x	1013
IX	0	450	563	94	2	x	x	x	x	1109
X	0	300	525	188	12	x	x	x	x	1025
XI	0	150	450	329	36	0	x	x	x	965
XII	0	0	338	319	83	3	x	x	x	743
XIII	0	0	188	291	165	12	0	x	x	656
XIV	0	0	0	235	163	33	1	x	x	432
XV	0	0	0	141	153	74	4	0	x	372
XVI	0	0	0	0	129	74	12	0	x	215
XVII	0	0	0	0	82	71	30	1	0	184
XVIII	0	0	0	0	0	63	30	4	0	97
XIX	0	0	0	0	0	41	29	12	0	83
XX	0	0	0	0	0	0	26	12	1	39
Total										12568

From the above table it results that after 19 years working we will dispose of 12 adult F7 adult females. This figure is valuable for the males as well. Then it is possible to move to the natural mating identifying the family of the rams and distributing the existing 83 females per families. Further the multiplication program must be completed with the selection of the wanted type of the former preserved breed.

The project used a conception rate of 50% per ewe/year. In order to reduce costs of the project fertility rate has to be increased to at least 100%. That is possible respecting the mentioned before principle recommending any artificial insemination session has to be completed by natural mating. In this case rams from the maternal breed must be used. In this respect it is very important the maternal breed to posse a genetically dominant qualitative trait allowing to recognizing the progeny of rams of the maternal breed.

Of course is more convenient to preserve embryo population which possesses diploid genomic information, a complete one. The depot of embryos needed to receive a sheep population of 4 families with about 30 females per family must be formatted from 1000 embryos (250 embryos per family), estimating a 24% conception rate after embryo transfer. At the same time it is not necessary to wait 14 years since obtaining the *"in situ"* sheep population.

Many hopes are related to the frequency of twins or triplets obtained from the receptors ewes, associated to small number of transfer embryos' lost. Al of these hopes aims to decrease the cost of applied MOET in selection or in commercial flocks.

We have to stress on the advantages of the full genotype of embryos in transmitting hereditary traits and on the efficiency of increasing the ovulation number in each estrus time as important factor to decreasing costs.

Some difficulties in developing reproduction biotechnologies with ewes result from the rather small body size of animals. It is possible to pass over these difficulties with good endoscopic equipment.

Chapter 5
VIRTUES AND SERVITUDES OF BREEDING BIOTECHNOLOGY IN SHEEP (Instead of conclusions)

Future of biotechnologies in sheep breeding

The older author of the present book had the opportunity in 1993 to attend the "Workshop on Biotechnology in Agriculture" organized at the International Center for Genetic Engineering and Biotechnology. Then the monitor of the Workshop, Mr. Decio Ripandelli, has said, (citing from memory) that "Biotechnology in Agriculture" is not a science and the lectures that will be presented will refer to the basic sciences of biotechnologies, the study object of the Centre. He said biotechnology is a set of techniques to obtaining biological products based on four sciences: Molecular Genetics, Gene Engineering, Protein Engineering and Bio Engineering". And so the Workshop will present further lectures from these four sciences. Students understood that Molecular Genetics searches how genetic information species is reproduced from one generation to the next one by DNA and how RNA transmits orders to the structures involved in growth of the bodies which support the genotypes of biological species commending protein synthesis. Gene Enginery, using discoveries from Molecular Genetics, may create genes with succession and repetition of codes able to command synthesis of single amino acid that produce wanted protein molecules. Protein Enginery gives the possibility to discover protein molecules' architecture and to synthesize pure proteins by succession of amino acid codes. Lesser was taught about Bio Enginery.

The Workshop was fabulous but we need to know more in order to understand how genetic information works. We have to know how epigenetic effect of genes (of proteins) acts as catalyzer commanding synthesis of sugars, lipids and of complex enzymes. Even more mysterious are the mechanisms commanding cell specialization during the ontogenetic development of animal or vegetal organisms and how architecture of organs and of organisms (ontogeny) is directed. All these concern Bioengineering.

Related to ontogenesis now days people speak about **stem cells**, about cells able to give other type of cell when are dividing. There is also a classification of cells from this point of view: totipotents (like the blastomeres or the umbilical cells), multipotents (embryonic cells), pluripotents (bone's medulla cells), monopotents (tissue cells) and nulipotents (neurons). How this process is commanded is mostly unknown. Craig Vernon the scientist claiming recently, in a TV presentation, success in artificial synthesis of cell, expressed the idea that nucleus of cell is acting as its software and the hardware is located in cell's protoplasm.

That is a very interesting idea. But how does work the nucleus software? May we suppose Autosomes (somatic chromosomes that are in pairs) are commanding gross protein synthesis for the soma growth meanwhile single Heterosomes (sexual chromosomes) are commanding the cells' differentiation and the organisms' development? It could be.

Some scientists seem to give positive answer to this question since they are looking for discovering in the Y mammalian chromosome the "testis determining factor" (TDF)[44] blocking ontogenesis of female reproductive organs in the genetically male embryos and determining male organs formation. Perhaps Y chromosome, a small one, acting single, is responsive as a whole for the secretion of enzymes acting successively in male reproductive apparatus development. May be the single X chromosome, a larger one, present in any embryo, doesn't matter of its sex (it was already demonstrated that in female genetic sex embryos in the 8 – 16 blastomeres stage one X chromosome of the pair is not replicated further remaining as the chromatin "drumstick"[45] permitting the sex diagnosis of embryos), acting on Autosomes will then command the female genital organs' development and also the whole body ontogeny in organisms of both sexes. The Y chromosome has the role of commanding the male sexual dimorphism and the Autosomes' pairs commanding organ growth.

This knowledge could be the first steps in Bio Enginery. If Enginery means *minding, projecting, constructing and using machinery, and by extension roads and bridges*, then Bio Enginery would mean *minding, projecting, creating and using live structures, using genomic bio techniques*. Genetics' Encyclopedic Dictionary [46] is giving 3 senses for the word "genome". In the first sense *genome is the totality of genes existing in a haploid set of chromosomes*. In the second sense *genome means the totality of genes of one group of linkage (chromosome)*

[44] Hafez, E.S.E.; Hafez, B. *Reproduction in Farm Animals.* seventh edition, Lippincott Williams Wilkins, Philadelphia, 2000
[45] Eldrige, F.E. *Cytogenetics of Livestock.* Avi Publishing Company Inc., 1985
[46] Maximilian, C.; Ioan, Doina Maria. *Dicţionar Enciclopedic de Genetică.* Editura Ştiinţifică şi Enciclopedică, Bucureşti, 1984

and in the third sense *genome is the totality of genes of a genotype (cell or organism)*. Oxford Dictionary[47] gives 2 definitions:

(1) *the haploid set of chromosomes of an organism* and

(2) *the complete set of genetic material of an organism.*

Out of these definitions we can conclude that Bio Engineering has to act with haploid or diploid groups of gene linkage.

At present animal farming have made progresses in reproducing artificial populations (by breeding), in reproducing artificial hybrids (by hybridization) in producing commercial genotypes (by crossbreeding) and in multiplying such results by reproduction biotechnologies like the ones presented in the former chapters of this book. Further successes are waited from Molecular Genetics, Gene Enginery, and Protein Enginery in creating *genomic biotechnologies* in the benefit of Bio Enginery which seems to be, at present, more a goal then a fundamental science.

Reproduction biotechnologies and *genomic biotechnologies* are virtues of good will creative human information concerning the sustainability of the future human society both from the food security and from the safety food parts. But as always information has two contrary sides. Opposite to good will creative human information bad will creative information can act. Example of bad will utilization of biotechnologies is bioterrorism, a very dangerous way of struggle between human communities presenting the risk of losing the control upon the used weapon. Therefore world or regional organizations in charge are afraid of servitudes of biotechnologies. Such documents are the "Council Directive of 23 April 1990 on the contained use of genetically modified micro-organisms (90/219/EEC)" and "Council Directive of 23 April 1990 on the deliberate realize into the environment of genetically modified micro-organisms (90/220/EEC)". But later on, of similar fears, Council of European Union forbids culture of GMO plants, as corn or soya been and all other ones. Recently they are rumors the same Council intends to ban farm animal cloning. Are these reasonable measures?

It is true that prokaryote biological species spread in nature is very difficult to be controlled since genetic species identity is based only on genotype structure and reproduction of their existing units (cells) admits transduction of DNA fragments between species[48]. Transduction is possible even in bacteria which dispose of cell membrane as the simplest tool of closed reproduction of

[47] *Concise Oxford English Dictionary.* eleventh edition, Oxford University Press, 2004
[48] Freifelder, D. *Microbial Genetics.* Jones and Bartlett Publishers, Boston, 1987

genotypes, protecting genetic species identity. Interdiction to free production of genetically modified viruses and bacteria is wholly justified. Extension of interdiction is justified to vegetal (*yeast, fungi or other*) and to one cell animal species (*Amoeba, Babesia, Coccidia or other)*, as well. The risk of DNA transduction in single cell eukaryote live beings is maintained since natural tools of closed reproduction have added to the membrane mechanisms of closed reproduction only mitosis division of cells.

In culture plants of superior genetic species closed reproduction is ensured by more strict means. They include nearby *clones* resulting from vegetative multiplication the rules of amphimixis of sexual gametes during the fertilization process. It is true that pollen granules are carried on long distances by wind or insects and natural hybrid plants are met in nature but the pollen granules have full male haploid genomes and transduction of free DNA sequences can't take place. GMO angiosperm plant culture forbidding because of safety food risk means an exaggerate prudence that has no justification. Many accidents were produced by natural mutations generating toxic species of mushrooms and no one from GMO kinds of angiosperm plants. No real servitude of plant GMO can be claimed.

Concerning farm animal genetic species we must say that natural mechanisms of closed reproduction are most severe than the ones of the angiosperm plants. High evolved genetic species strongly defeat their identity. There are at least 6 molecular mechanisms closing reproduction in farm animal genetic species, known up to now. These are: *Zona Pellucida Reaction*, the *Vitellin Membrane Block*, the *Karyotype*, the *Allele Genes' Complimentary*, the *Major Histocompatibility Complex* and the *Maternal Recognition of Pregnancy*.[49] In addition the *sexual behavior* of species disposing of brain cognition information strengthens the power of closed reproduction natural mechanism[50]. We don't know any case of hybrid between genetic species in nature. Then which is the reason to forbid research concerning the cloning of farm animals?

Farm animal cloning presents no risk from food security or for safety food. On contrary it might help food security with better conversion of food production resources and produce not only safety food but medicine food. Already transgenesis in farm animal zygote made possible to have non immuno reactive

---

[49] Paraschivescu, M. *Molecular mechanisms of closed reproduction in mammals farm animals.* Lucrări Ştiinţifice, seria Zootehnie, volum 45, Editura Ion Ionescu de la Brad, Iaşi, 2002
[50] Paraschivescu, M.Th.; Bogdan, A.T.; Paraschivescu, M.; Tobă, G.F.; Stan, Simona *Biodiversity in farm animals: sources, using, conservation.* Lucrări ştiinţifice, Seria D vol.LII, U.S.A.M.V. Bucureşti 2009; pag.89-95

human insulin (HI) or to master the hamster's *tissue plasmino activator* (TPA) from transgenic cows or ewes. These are virtues. Servitudes of genomic biotechnologies with farm animals are the difficulties to obtaining the wanted transgenic organisms and to multiplying them. That determines very high costs of transgenic animals and of their clones.

Recent progress in genome's study evolved the idea of artificial selection based on SNIPs panel of parental pairs. We think this is only a hope which is not fully justified. People thinking this way ignore the phenomenon of meiosis present in gameto genesis. When meiosis takes place chromosome splitting in ovocit or spermatocit distribute equally the genes as number, but not the number of single nucleotides. SNIPs will differ from gamete to gamete. That explains why quantitative traits of breeds can be increased from generation to generation by artificial selection. Or may be some time one or another gene suffer mutation or imprinting. There is no guaranty such phenomenon could be discovered by SNIPs.

On the other hand SNIPs don't offer information about body architecture making up the *type of animal*. Or body type has great importance in the phenotype evaluation of farm animals for breeding new generations. In the current practice evaluation of *type has to guaranty the resistance of the body to the effort imposed by the genotype.* The best understanding of this question pertains to American breeders of dairy cows. They evaluate the *Stature (frame)* prizing large animals but not heavy, in order to have animals able to eat much as basis for high milk production. They appreciate the *Support (legs)* because a large body is heavy and requires strong bones and joints. Great attention is paid to the ankles' angle and to the form of the hoofs. *Suspension* of the inner organs to the backbone (spinal column) is estimated considering the direction of the superior line of the body. It must be strait and horizontally directed. Great attention is paid to the *Udder attachment,* which is indicated by the *firmness of the cleft* (the median udder ligament) together with the *quarters' symmetry, gland vasculature* and *teats' sizes.* No one of these traits can be appreciated through SNIPs analysis. But SNIPs offer sure information about identity of genotypes and about animals' genealogy. Still now there is no restriction in studying farm animal genomes.

May be banning mammals cloning has bioethical reasons. The fear of extending cloning procedures from farm animal to human beings could be such a reason. Cloning of humans is a bad matter not only from ethical point of view but it is bad from the medical point of view as well. Humans understood along the time the misfortune giving by reducing intra species variability by incest. Cloning of human genotypes could be worse since it will minimize the populations' variability extremely. Banning of cloning human beings has reason and must be sustained. But there is no need to legally forbid animal farm cloning. On the other hand there are not reasons genomic biotechnologies with transgenic animals and clones to enter farming soon because of costs. Few hopes are for the future, as well. Perhaps they will enter in pharmaceutical industry, but that isn't bad at wall.

Biotechnologies with farm animals present no servitudes from biotechnical point of view. Let international scientifically organizations like *International Embryo Transfer Society, International Office for Epizooties* or *World Health Organization* to monitor research activity genetics, in farming or in veterinary medicine. Political organizations like Organization of United Nations or European Union Council have to solve other very difficult questions as Human Demographic Increment, Global Heating of the Earth planet or the future Cultural Globalization of the World. Solutions to this kind of questions pertain to politics. They will be successfully if the equity for all human communities from the smallest to the largest ones will be solved in any respects.

Future of biodiversity in sheep farming

Intensive sheep farming must become more and more extended. Specialized breeds for lean mutton or for milk production will be bred for this system. Concerning mutton breeds two lambing per year is a target to be hit. In milking sheep breeds it is of interest to suppress seasonal anestrous and to have as long lactation as to covering 2/3 of pregnancy. This is a very difficult target but nevertheless a possible one.

The answer to the question how the commercial quality of the Karakul pelts is genetically correlated to the milk production ability of use and to the body size of the lamb's parents, or to the meaty traits of adult animal carcasses will decide if the Karakul breed responds to intensive farming.

Extensive sheep farming will continue to exist in poor vegetation areas. In dry, warm climate areas thin wool breeds will be preferred. In dry cold areas with two contrast season concerning feeding resources pelts breeds are recommended. On high alpine pastures thick wool, light ewes are most suitable.

Sheep biodiversity must be sustained by single Breed Associations controlling its closed breeding on a Flock Book base. Uncontrolled crossbreeding is the main cause of losing the genetic species biodiversity and a high risk for the flocks' health, including the scrappy disease. Preservation of breeds in critical states will prefer *in situ* preservation of diploid genomic structures.

Artificial insemination as reproduction system will be practically applied only with blind insemination and Embryo transfer will be associated to valuable genotypes only.

In vitro fertilization will be used to create transgenic organisms and their clones in order to produce medicines. Such procedures are too expensive for producing food or other domestic goods.

There are plenty of undemonstrative spare outputs in sheep breeding and sheep farming to be disclosed by biotechnologies.

BIBLIOGRAPHY

1. **BARI, F.; KHALIDB, M.; HARESIGN, W.** *Factors affecting the survival of sheep embryos after transfer within a MOET program.* Theriogenology 59, 2003

2. **DINU, Cristina; PARASCHIVESCU, Marcel; CAPROȘU, V.** *Durata sezonului de montă la oile Corriedale și implicațiile acesteia în reproducție.* Zilele Cercetării Științifice, ICPCOC Palas, 1994

3. **DINU, Cristina; PARASCHIVESCU, M.; SZABO, I.** *Controlul situației ginecologice în sezonul de montă prin prostaglandine, la oile Corriedale.* Analele IBNA, vol.XVIII, 1995

4. **ELDRIGE, F.E.** *Cytogenetics of Livestock.* Avi Publishing Company Inc., 1985

5. **FREIFELDER, David.** *Microbial Genetics.* Jones and Bartlett Publishers, Boston, 1987

6. **FURTUNESCU, Alexandru.** *Zootehnie Generală.* vol.I, Editura Agrosilvică de Stat, București, 1958

7. **GROZA, Ioan Ștefan.** *Actualități și perspective în biotehnologia transferului de embrioni la specia ovină.* Editura Ceres, București, 1996

8. **HARTL, Daniel L.; FREIFELDER, David; SNYDER, Leon.** *Basic Genetics.* Johnes and Bartlett Publishers Boston Portola Valley, 1988

9. **HAFEZ, Elsayed Saad Eldin.** *Reproduction in Farm Animals.* Lea & Febiger, Philadelphia, 1962

10. **HAFEZ, Elsayed Saad Eldin.; HAFEZ, B.** *Reproduction in Farm Animals.* seventh edition, Lippincott Williams Wilkins, Philadelphia, 2000

11. **KHOBOSO, Christina Lehloenya.** *Multiple Ovulation and Embryo Transfer in Goats.* PhD thesis, 2008

12. **LAMOND, D.R.** *Animal Breeding Abstract.* 32 p., No.3, 1964

13. **MATEESCU, Raluca.** *Marker Assisted Selection in Animal Breeding.* Training course at Animal Biology and Nutrition Institute, Bucharest, Romania, 2011

14. **MAXIMILIAN, C.; IOAN, Doina Maria.** *Dicționar Enciclopedic de Genetică.* Editura Științifică și Enciclopedică, București, 1984

15. **MOCANU, Viorel; PARASCHIVESCU, Marcel and alii.** *Spermatozoa capacitation conditioning in vitro fertilization.* Arhiva Zootehnică IBNA, 1989

16. **MOOR, R.M.; CLARK, A.J.** *Molecular Embryology.* Report for 1989-1990, Institute of Animal Physiology and Genetics Research, Cambridge and Edinburgh Research Stations

17. **OȚEL, Vasile; PARASCHIVESCU, Marcel; MIHĂILESCU, Constantin.** *Fertilitatea și Infertilitatea la Animalele de Fermă,* Editura Agrosilvică, București, 1967

18. **OȚEL, Vasile; HARSHIANU, A.; PARASCHIVESCU, Marcel.** *Sincronizarea estrului la ovine I.* Lucrări științifice ale ICZ vol.XXIV, București, 1966

19. **OȚEL, Vasile; PARASCHIVESCU, Marcel; PETRIA, I.** *Sincronizarea estrului la ovine II.* Lucrări științifice ale ICZ vol.XXV, 1967

20. **PARAIPAN, Virgil.** *Hormonoterapia la Animalele Domestice.* Editura Agrosilvică, 1982

21. **PARASCHIVESCU, Marcel.** *Contribuții la cunoașterea și îmbunătățirea procesului tehnologic din centrele mari de însămânțări artificiale la oi.* PhD Thesis, Veterinary Medicine Faculty, Bucharest, Romania, 1963

22. **PARASCHIVESCU, Marcel.** *Reproducția la Ovine,* Editura Agrosilvică, 1969

23. **PARASCHIVESCU, Marcel.** *Molecular mechanisms of closed reproduction in mammals farm animals.* Lucrări Științifice, seria Zootehnie, volum 45, Editura Ion Ionescu de la Brad, Iași, 2002

24. **PARASCHIVESCU, Marcel.** *Biodiversity in Farm Animals: Sources, Using, Conservation.* Scientific Papers, D series, volume LII, USAMV Bucharest, 2009

25. **PARASCHIVESCU, Marcel.** *Gnosis foundation of biological diversity.* Report at Rumanian Academy of Agriculture and Forestry Sciences, June 2011

26. **PARASCHIVESCU, Marcel; DINU, Cristina; POPA, I.** *Efectul prostaglandinei asupra corpului galben de călduri și corpului galben de gestație la oile Țurcană.* Analele IBNA, vol.XVII, 1995

27. **PARASCHIVESCU, Marcel; GHERCIU, Mihaela; DINU, Cristina; NIȚULESCU, Aneta; MURAT, I.** *Observații privind desfășurarea reproducției prin montă naturală.* Analele IBNA, vol.XVI, 1993

28. **PARASCHIVESCU, Marcel; IONĂȘESCU, L.** *Utilization of "Synchromate" for the synchronization of heat in sheep mating season.* G.D.Searle London, 1967

29. **PARASCHIVESCU, Marcel; PARASCHIVESCU, Marcel Theodor.** *Psychic stress and animal welfare in dairy cattle production.* Scientific papers C series volumul LVIII (3), F.M.V.Bucureşti, 2012

30. **PARASCHIVESCU, Marcel; PARASCHIVESCU, Marcel Theodor; BOGDAN, Alexandru T.; STAN, Simona.** *Animal rights and their welfare in concept, laws, actions.* Simpozionul cu tema „Contribuţii ale cercetării ştiinţifice la progresul medicinii veterinare" F.M.V.Bucureşti Scientific papers C series volumul LVII(1), 2011

31. **PARASCHIVESCU, Marcel; MOCANU, Viorel; PARASCHIVESCU, Maria.** *Hatchery Farm in Dairy Cattle Breeding.* Veterinary Medicine Society, Open discussion upon against diseases protection, 1989

32. **PARASCHIVESCU, Marcel; URSESCU, Alexandru.** *Influenţarea vieţii sexuale la ovine în sezonul de primăvară prin tratamente hormonale.* Lucrările Congresului Internaţional de Biologie a Reproducţiei, Moscova, 1966

33. **PARASCHIVESCU, Marcel; URSESCU, Alexandru.** *Ovarian stimulation in sheep out of the estrus season.* G.D.Searle London 68, 1967

34. **PARASCHIVESCU, Marcel; URSESCU, Alexandru.** *Sincronizarea estrului la ovine III. Frecvenţa stărilor anestrale.* Revista de Zootehnie şi Medicină Veterinară nr.10, 1968

35. **PARASCHIVESCU, Marcel; URSESCU, Alexandru.** *Sincronizarea estrului la ovine IV. Durata progesteronemiei induse şi efectul gonadotrofinelor.* Revista de Zootehnie şi Medicină Veterinară, nr.11, 1969

36. **PARASCHIVESCU, Marcel; URSESCU, Alexandru.** *Sincronizarea estrului la ovine V. Frecvenţa stărilor anestrale.* Revista de Zootehnie şi Medicină Veterinară nr.10, 1970

37. **PARASCHIVESCU, Marcel; URSESCU, Alexandru; LEPĂDATU, C.** *Sincronizarea estrului la ovine III.* Revista de Zootehnie şi Medicină Veterinară, nr.12, Consiliul Superior al Agriculturii, 1968

38. **PARASCHIVESCU, Marcel; VLAD, C.; CONSTANTINESCU, L.; PĂTRAŞCU, Mircea.** *Rezultate ale reproducţiei intensive îndelungate la ovine.* Lucrările seminarului de Reproducţie, Patologia Reproducţiei şi Boli Neo-natale. Universitatea Agricolă Cluj, 1984

39. **PARASCHIVESCU, Marcel Theodor.** *Studiu de proiect privind înfiinţarea unei ferme MOET cu circuit deschis.* Teză de Doctorat, U.S.A.M.V.Bucureşti, 2002

40. **PARASCHIVESCU, Marcel Theodor; BOGDAN, Alexandru T.; PARASCHIVESCU, Marcel; TOBĂ, George Florea; STAN, Simona.** *Biodiversity in farm animals: sources, using, conservation.* Lucrări ştiinţifice, Seria D vol.LII, U.S.A.M.V. Bucureşti, 2009

41. **PARASCHIVESCU, Marcel Theodor; BOGDAN, Alexandru T.; PARASCHIVESCU, Marcel; IPATE, Iudith, TOBĂ, George Florea.** *Degrees of extensin risk in farm animal breeds.* Buletin Agriculture, vol.67 (2), USAMV Cluj-Napoca, 2010

42. **PARASCHIVESCU, Marcel Theodor; PARASCHIVESCU, Marcel; CONSTANTINESCU, Dan.** *Superioritatea folosirii embrio-transferului în transferarea unor populaţii de vite.* Lucrări ştiinţifice, seria Zootehnie, volum 65, Editura Ion Ionescu de la Brad, Iaşi, 2002

43. **PARASCHIVESCU, Marcel Theodor; PARASCHIVESCU, Marcel; BOGDAN, Alexandru T.; TOBĂ, George Florea; SANDU, Mariana; IPATE, Judith; STAN, Simona; DOBRE, Dana.** *Some aspects of farm animal biodiversity formation on Romania's actual teritory.* DAGENE, Hunedoara, 2010

44. **PARASCHIVESCU, Marcel Theodor; ŞONEA, Alexandru; BOGDAN, Alexandru T.; PARASCHIVESCU, Marcel; TOBĂ, George Florea.** *Essay on estimation of undemonstrative spare outputs disclosed by reproduction biotechnologies in sheep breeding.* Simpozionul "Agriculture for Life, Life for Agriculture", University of Agronomic Sciences and Veterinary Medicine of Bucharest, Romania, Scientific papers series D. Animal science vol.LV 2012

45. **REIK, W.; HOWLETT, S.K.; SURANI, M.A.H.** *Imprinting and genetic disease.* Report for 1989-1990, Institute of Animal Physiology and Genetics Research, Cambridge and Edinburgh Research Stations, 1991

46. **ROBERTSON, Edwin.** *Estrus Syinchronization Programs that Work.* Harrogate Genetics International, Harrogate, Tennessee, 1999

47. **ROWSON, L.E.A.; MOOR, R.M.** Embryo transfer in the sheep: the significance of synchronizing oestrus in the donor and recipient animal; Journal of Reproduction and Fertility 11, 196634. Pawson, H.C. *Robert Bakewell. Pioneer livestock breeder.* London: Crosby Lockwood & Son, Ltd, 1957

48. **VOICU, Rita; CAPROŞU, A.; PARASCHIVESCU, Marcel; GHIŢĂ, Elena.** *Efectul selecţiei direcţionale consecutiv procedeelor de ameliorare în rasă curată a oilor Corriedale.* Anale IBNA, volum XVI, 1993

49. **WILLADSEN, S.M.; POLGE, C.; ROWSON, L.E.A.; MOOR, R.M.** *Deep freezing of sheep embryos.* Journal of Reproduction and Fertility 46, 1976

50. **ZAMFIRESCU, Stela; ȘONEA, Alexandru.** *Biotehnologii de Reproducere la Rumegătoarele Mici.* ISBN: 973-644-113-X, Editura ExPonto, 2004

51. *** *Definitions of Terms used in Agricultural Business Management.* Second edition, Ministry of Agriculture, Fisheries and Food, 1977

52. *** *Council Directive of 23 April 1990 on the contained use of genetically modified micro-organisms* (90/219/EEC)"

53. *** *Council Directive of 23 April 1990 on the deliberate realize into the environment of genetically modified micro-organisms* (90/220/EEC)".

54. *** *International Embryo Transfer Society.* Manual of the International Embryo Transfer Society, 2nd ed. (D.A. Stringfellow and S.M. Seidel, ed.). IETS, Champaign, IL, USA, 1990

55. *** *Convention for biological biodiversity.* Rio de Janeiro, 1992

56. *** *Office Internationale des Epizooties. Section 3.2. "Collection of semen",* 2000

57. *** *Concise Oxford English Dictionary.* Eleventh edition, Oxford University Press, 2004

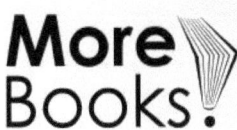
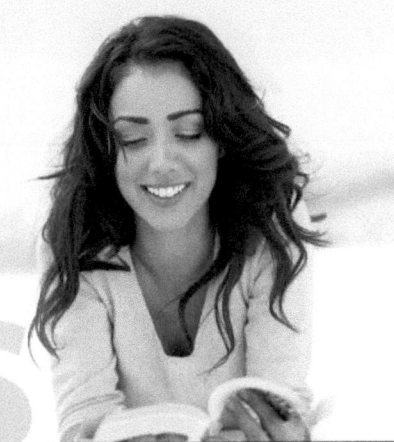

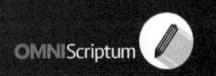

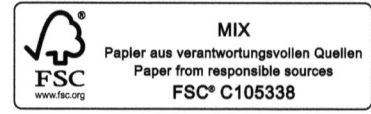
Printed by Books on Demand GmbH, Norderstedt / Germany